EATING HABITS FOR HEALTHY SKIN

9 EATING HABITS TO HELP YOUR ACNE, ECZEMA OR PSORIASIS

CLAIRE HAMILTON

Eating Habits for Healthy Skin

Copyright © Claire Hamilton 2020

ISBN: 978-1-8381777-0-6
Published by TLC Publications Ltd

CONTENTS

YOUR FREE RESOURCES

To help you get the most out of this book, download your book bonuses from

www.thelifestylecircle.com/bookbonuses

You'll find a collection of free printables to help you build sustainable healthy habits.

I don't believe your lifestyle has caused your skin issues. The cause is likely to be far more complex. But I do believe lifestyle is an essential element of healing the skin.

These bonuses will help you to start and stick with your new eating habits for your best skin.

Book Bonuses Downloads

- Action steps as a checklist
- Your first steps printable
- Overcoming obstacles printable
- 30 fruit and vegetables tracker
- Meal planner template
- Mindful eating diary template
- Month to view calendar
- Your lifestyle circle printable
- A guide to skin types
- A guide to using an emollient

Download from www.thelifestylecircle.com/bookbonuses

INTRODUCTION

> Food isn't like medicine, it is medicine, and it's our number one tool for creating the vibrant health we deserve.
>
> Mark Hyman, M.D

People say you should write the book you always wanted to read. This book is it. But I didn't write it for me. I wrote it for the girl with the long brown hair that I see walking to school in the mornings. Her acne reminds me of mine. I see her long sleeves and thick tights, regardless of the weather, and wonder if she's hiding her skin for the same reasons that I hid mine.

When I struggled with acne, eczema, and psoriasis, it was the early 1990s. I didn't have the Internet, and I didn't know anyone else who suffered with their skin. On the plus side, I couldn't spend hours online looking for weird and wonderful cures, but it was very isolating. I looked around me and saw no one who looked like me or understood what I was going through.

Now I see lots of people who are going through the same thing. If you're one of these people, then this book is for you too. But I also see people making the same mistakes I did. Cutting things out of their diets, possibly unnecessarily, and spending a fortune on skincare programs that did nothing but exacerbate my skin issues. I see people believing that medication to manage the symptoms is the only way forward, and I see my desperation from the past reflected in their words.

I work with a community of people through my website www.thelifestylecircle.com to help them make lifestyle changes to get their best skin. I help people to make new, healthier habits that they can maintain long term.

There are many ways to heal the skin. I wrote this book to tell others struggling with their skin what worked for me. I recognise that what worked for me might not work for everyone. But it will undoubtedly work for some people. If it takes a few years off the search for your solution, then I'm happy. The more we talk about what's working for us, the fewer people who will suffer from these life-affecting skin conditions.

I struggled for 10 years with my skin when only a few simple tweaks to my diet were needed. These tweaks, though simple, took time for me to figure out and to implement.

The world of healthy eating is cluttered with fad diets and conflicting viewpoints. There's lots of information on weight loss, heart health, blood pressure, and diabetes, but it's still rare to find a book that talks specifically about what we eat and the health of our skin.

Change can be hard, but it's even harder changing something you've probably been doing the same way all of your life – your eating habits.

If you're suffering from acne, eczema, or psoriasis, you might also suffer from irritable bowel syndrome, headaches, and sinus issues. I know this because I had these symptoms too. And as you'll discover, there's a good chance that many of your symptoms are linked.

Some of these conditions are so commonplace that we've begun to think of them as normal. They're not. As my skin cleared, all of these other health conditions eased or disappeared too. You don't need to put up with these things every day.

Despite being told many times that my skin conditions were not related to my diet, I knew that couldn't be true. What I was eating must have had some connection to the state of my skin.

Let me get the necessary disclaimer out of the way. This book is not nutritional advice, nor is it a diet plan giving you meal plans and shopping lists. It's a book about changing your eating *habits*, which are fundamental to how healthy you, and your skin, are.

We all know eating an apple is better for us than eating a cake. We don't need a book to tell us that. But having knowledge and applying knowledge are two different things.

Through this book, I will teach you a system to apply what you already know to be true healthy eating practices.

I've created your action plan. I've developed the tools you need and thought about how to overcome the obstacles that will inevitably crop up. All you need to do is follow along with this book, and you will change your eating habits for the better. Changing my eating habits was key to relieving my acne, eczema, and psoriasis. Changing your eating habits might finally be the thing that brings you relief too.

My goal with this book is to provide you with a quick read, actionable advice, and tools you can start using today.

I don't want to take you through a temporary program that doesn't give you lasting results. I want to inspire a permanent life change for you.

ABOUT THIS BOOK

In this book, we'll go through why eating vegetables and drinking water is essential to eating well, and why they helped me heal my skin. Please don't be put off by how simple that sounds. You might think it seems too simple to work. But I promise you it does work.

I will share some leading research with you to change the way you think about what you put on your plate.

We'll look at why our habits are vital to improving our health, and why it's easier than we think to change our habits by borrowing the techniques we, as parents, use every day to teach our children.

You'll get nine new habits to nurture to get you eating well for life.

We'll look at the obstacles that might stop you from making changes. You'll learn how to review any other obstacles that might crop up for you. I'll also give you specific solutions to overcome the most common obstacles, so you have everything you need to take action and transform your health.

How this book breaks down:

> **Part 1:** Our skin – what it is and why some of us get issues.

> **Part 2:** What is a healthy diet and the gut skin connection.

> **Part 3:** Exercises to get you started on the journey to your best skin.

> **Part 4:** The nine eating habits for healthy skin.

> **Part 5:** Frequently asked questions.

> **Part 6:** How to make changing your habits as easy as possible.

> **Part 7:** Overcoming common obstacles to change.

> **Part 8:** Accountability and sticking to your new habits.

> **Part 9:** Conclusion and next steps for you to start today.

The focus of this book is your eating habits. Hands down, changing my eating habits had the most dramatic shift for me. But I see lifestyle as wider than food.

A healthy lifestyle means focusing on my food choices, my mind, my body, and my environment. When I have a sense of balance in those areas, I'm happier, healthier, and my skin stays in good condition. When I'm out of alignment in any of those areas, I don't feel at my healthiest.

Additional resources

There are three additional resources I'll refer you to at the end of this book to help you get your best skin quicker.

1. **Your lifestyle circle exercise.** When we give ourselves the space to listen to our bodies, we know what changes we need to make to improve our health. This resource will guide you through other key areas of your life to identify any other aspects of your lifestyle that need a bit of TLC.

2. **A guide to skin types.** When it came to my acne, eating well had a dramatic effect. But figuring out my true skin type was the final piece of the puzzle. Spoiler alert – acne-prone skin is not a skin type. This guide will show you why your skincare products might be doing more harm than good and what to do instead.

3. **A guide to using an emollient.** Emollients are still one of the main treatments prescribed for eczema and psoriasis. In this guide, I share the technique for applying an emollient that my doctor taught me. After years of using emollients with little effect, this is the technique that made a difference.

HOW TO USE THIS BOOK

Reading this book will not help your skin. Taking action on what you read will.

Please don't make this a book you read then do nothing with. It's useful information, but it's also an action plan. It's easy to follow steps that will dramatically improve your health with as little effort as possible. But it will still require some effort.

Dip in and out of this book as often as you need to. Coming back to it a few times will refresh your memory, spark new ideas, and help you see where you might need to make tweaks to your actions.

Healing your skin is not a one-time thing. It's a process.

I suggest you review where you are at different points throughout the year to check on how you're feeling and where you need extra effort to get the best results.

Don't be put off by the thought of work. I've done my best to make it as easy as possible for you.

The idea behind this book is not for you to change your whole routine. That will overwhelm you, and you won't get the results you want.

This book will instead ask you to add things to your current diet and routine. It will focus on small steps that build momentum over time and lead to lasting changes to your habits.

Some people can make sudden and dramatic changes, many of us can't, particularly when it comes to our eating habits. We decide to cut the crap from our diets, but three days and a chocolate binge later, we wind up right back where we started and feeling pretty miserable.

With a clear system and a set of tools at your disposal, anyone can make lasting changes to their habits.

One thing at a time

Before we get stuck in, just a quick word on doing one thing at a time. People who change their health rarely do only one thing despite what they say.

Kale, celery juice, yoga, vitamin C serum, or whatever else has been recommended to you will not heal your skin. They all have their benefits, but they will have little effect on their own.

People who start eating better will eat more vegetables and drink more water. But they're also likely to reduce their sugar intake, sleep better and be more conscious of how much they're moving throughout the day.

The Institute of Integrative Nutrition (IIN) calls this 'crowding out'. Essentially, by adding goodness to your diet, there's less room for the foods that aren't serving your health.

The more you become conscious of how healthy your plate looks, the more aware you become of other areas of your health. You'll find yourself becoming more aware of how much exercise you're doing, how much sleep you're getting, and how you feel on particular days and after eating certain foods.

The more progress you make with your new eating habits, the more positive you'll become about your health. My advice is to focus on using the tools to get you in the habit of eating well. Don't worry about trying to change too many other habits at the same time.

If you notice you've been sitting down for hours, get up and move around. If you're tired and would benefit from an early night, go ahead and have one. But don't stress about having to move more or having to sleep more. Slow and steady does it. These other things will all come in time.

MY STORY

I was about 13 years old and home sick from school when there was a knock at my front door. I opened it to someone who told me they were the truant officer. I remember the nerves in my stomach and the flush on my cheeks. Gone were the days of primary school and perfect attendance. Now I was in high school, and I was sick for a few days every month for 18 months.

I had recurring tonsillitis and was drugged up on antibiotics. It was during this time that my skin broke out. It started with psoriasis, which is an autoimmune disease that caused large patches of raised, scaly skin to form on my forearms and lower legs. Acne followed, then eczema.

When I first asked for help to deal with my skin, I was told it was bad luck, and I would grow out of it. I was given a thick yellow cream to coat my legs with, ointments to bathe in, steroid creams, more antibiotics, and the contraceptive pill. Nothing worked. My skin was awful, and my self-esteem plummeted.

My gut wasn't happy either. I was diagnosed with irritable bowel syndrome (IBS) that gave me excruciating cramps in my stomach almost every day. I had heartburn, headaches, and frequent bouts of sinusitis.

I saw specialists, including GPs, dermatologists, gastroenterologists, nutritionists, Chinese medicine practitioners, and alternative health professionals.

This was all happening in the early 1990s. Years later, I learned about the gut skin connection and realised that my symptoms were all linked. But at that time there was no suggestion of this. I had no access to the Internet, and it wasn't what it is today. The volume of information wasn't there, and this was in an era where antibiotics were still prescribed for the common cold.

I asked my doctor if there was a connection to the food I was eating. He assured me there was no link between diet and skin conditions but agreed to test me for a dairy intolerance anyway to see if that might be responsible for my gut issues. The test came back negative.

Alongside the treatments from my doctor, I had been trying to heal my acne from the outside. I cleansed, toned and moisturised my skin twice a day and continued to use the prescription creams.

I tried skincare products for acne-prone skin that you can buy on the high street. I tried the premium brands and specialist brands that you could only buy online. I was at university and waitressing part-time. My skincare regime was more than I could afford!

The premium brands and the specialist treatment programs irritated my skin. My skin was more inflamed than ever, red, sore, and flaky. I switched to tea tree products. My skin calmed down, but it did nothing to heal my acne.

A Chinese Medicine practitioner gave me acupuncture and a big bag of dried plants to make into a tonic. I soaked the plants in water until it turned into a dark brown liquid. It looked and smelled revolting, like something you'd find in a clogged drain. In desperation, I drank it down. It didn't work. I also tried cutting a variety of foods out of my diet to see if I could pinpoint anything that was causing my skin to flare-up.

I wore thick tights and long sleeves at school to hide my psoriasis. When we had swimming for PE, I was always in trouble for "forgetting" my swimsuit. I hated summer. I live in Scotland where the weather is not exactly tropical, but you still sweat too much if you're wearing jeans and long sleeves.

I'd gone from school to university and then the workplace with skin conditions. I'd accepted that my skin was always going to be an issue for me, and there was nothing I could do about it. I kept on using skincare for acne-prone skin and emollients for my eczema and psoriasis in an attempt to calm my skin down while realising it was never going to fix the problem. I gave up. I couldn't think of anything else to try.

Gut trouble

Meanwhile, my IBS continued to cause me problems. None of the treatments various doctors had given me worked. I would only schedule meetings at work in the mornings because I knew the afternoons were going to be difficult for me. I would get terrible stomach cramps almost every afternoon. Sometimes I would have to hide out in the toilets just holding my stomach in agony until they passed.

On occasion, they would be so bad I would be writhing in pain and sweating so much I would have to lie on a tiled floor just to cool down.

I now had the Internet and spent hours googling IBS. It didn't help. All I could find was that no one was sure how or why people got IBS. I was prescribed antispasmodics to calm my insides down. It was thought the pain was coming from spasms in some part of my bowel and medication to stop the spasms would reduce the pain.

Although I hadn't had great experiences with cutting foods out of my diet for my skin, I suspected there was a link between what I was eating and my IBS.

I paid for private food intolerance testing. The test results came back with a list of 19 foods that my blood showed a reaction to including dairy, beef, mushrooms, coffee, wheat, lentils, salmon, and kiwi fruit.

As part of the testing package, I worked with a nutritionist for two months. I ditched dairy and switched to soya milk and soy-based butter. I ate gluten-free bread and pasta and eliminated all of the foods that blood tests showed my body was reacting to.

I avoided going out to eat and turned down invitations from friends because I knew I would find it challenging to maintain my restricted diet. I also didn't want to deal with the questions from friends and family about my 'faddy diet'.

I didn't see any improvements in that period. While writing

this book, I pulled out the food diary I had been given at the time. I was asked to track my food as well as how I felt each day using a rating of 1 – 5, with 1 being 'worse' and 5 being 'excellent'. On every day except one, I rated myself as either 1 'worse' or 2 'same as before'.

In one of my final sessions with the nutritionist, I complained that I wasn't seeing any improvements. He told me soya could have the same effect on people as dairy so I should try switching to rice milk instead.

I felt completely dejected. Like the last two months had been a complete waste of time, and I would have to start all over again.

I switched to rice milk then eventually to almond milk. I started rating myself as 'same as before' rather than 'worse' not long after the switch.

Another interesting feature of my food diary at that time was just how little fruit and vegetables I ate. My discussions with the nutritionist focused on whether or not I was managing to eliminate my "problem foods". There were no conversations about increasing the amount of fruit and vegetables I was eating or aiming for greater variety. Each week of my food diary looked pretty much the same as the one before.

My sessions with the nutritionist ended, and I felt I hadn't made any progress.

The last straw

The last straw for me was another visit to my GP about my IBS.

I asked my doctor what else we could try. He gave me a prescription for a different set of pills. He explained that the pills treat depression, but they could have a positive impact on IBS. I took the prescription, got in my car and drove home. I did not stop at the pharmacy, and I never picked up that prescription. I had no intention of taking pills designed to mess with the chemicals in my brain when I didn't need them.

I had already given up trying to heal my skin, and now I had to give up trying to fix my IBS. I believed the doctors that these were just conditions I would have to live with. But for some reason, I wasn't downhearted.

I didn't want to spend the rest of my life feeling ill and taking medication. This was such a pivotal moment for me that I can still picture my doctor's office and the car park from which I drove away. I decided that day to accept my issues and focus instead on becoming the healthiest version of myself, even if I wasn't yet clear how to do this.

I wasn't overweight, I exercised, albeit sporadically, and I didn't eat a lot of junk food. But there's always room for improvement. It was at a friend's party when I stumbled across something that would change my eating habits for life and give me what I needed to heal my skin.

The path to good health

At the party, I grabbed a plate from the end of the buffet table. It was the usual table of party food: sausage rolls, sandwiches, crisps, chips, and cake. The visual struck me because it was all so beige. I couldn't get the image out of my mind, and it made me reflect on my diet.

I was in a food rut, I realised, with beige meals that centred on bread and pasta.

I tried to eat the recommended five portions of fruit and vegetables a day. I regularly ate bananas, apples, peas, sweetcorn, and tomatoes. But that was it. There was little variety.

I went on a mission to Banish the Beige from my diet. I still ate toast and pasta, but I made much more effort to add colour to my meals. It wasn't as difficult as I thought it might be and I still ate lots of chocolate.

This small change led to the other habit changes in this book, and a funny thing happened. My skin cleared up quite dramatically, and I saw lots of other improvements in my health.

I stood at the mirror one morning, grabbed a tube of concealer and dabbed some on to my finger. This had been my routine for 10 years. I looked into the mirror and realised that there was nothing to cover on my face. No blemishes, spots, or inflamed skin.

Sharing my story

My daughter suffered from baby eczema on her neck and torso when she was nine months old. I took her to the doctor who confirmed it was eczema. He gave us a prescription for hydrocortisone cream.

I questioned the doctor about what may be causing her eczema. I asked if it might be her bathing products or diet-related, even though she'd barely begun to eat solid foods. He said there was no link between diet and eczema, some babies just get it, and the only way to deal with it is to use a cream to help reduce the itch.

I picked up the cream from the pharmacy. I looked at her sore, broken skin and read the patient information leaflet inside the box. *Steroid cream...do not use on broken or infected skin...repeated use can cause skin thinning.*

That was when I realised we'd gone a whole generation, and nothing had changed about how we treat eczema.

I put the cream back in the box and decided to try to help my daughter by using what had worked for me.

I prepared her weaning foods with a wide variety of fruit and vegetables. I changed her bath products, baby wipes and used coconut oil to moisturise her skin, morning and night.

After two weeks, her eczema was gone.

I realised my results were not a fluke. They were repeatable, and other people could benefit from our experiences. I launched www.thelifestylecircle.com and began sharing what I was learning.

Food has the most significant influence on my skin. For my daughter, it's skincare products.

We know from our experience over the years that her skin is very reactive to products. If we try something new, some-times her skin is fine, and other times it will itch. We stop using anything that makes her skin itch and within a day or so her skin has settled down. She's at school now, and her eczema has never come back.

Is my health perfect? No. But not struggling with acne,

eczema, and psoriasis has been truly life-changing for me. These conditions are physically painful and emotionally draining. They are with you every single day of your life.

Even now, whenever someone comments on how good my skin is, my standard response is 'oh it wasn't always like this'. It's never just 'thank you'. Note to self, just say thank you next time.

Why am I qualified to talk about acne, eczema and psoriasis?

There's no one more qualified to talk about skin issues than someone that's suffered from them. People who haven't struggled with their skin tend to think acne is a few spots, eczema is a bit of an itch, and psoriasis is unsightly.

Only someone that's had a skin condition understands how invasive it is to all areas of your life.

You might hold yourself back from doing what you want to do because of your skin. You put limitations in place because of the physical or emotional pain you feel. You feel helpless, as though your body is at war with itself, and there's nothing you can do about it.

Taking charge of my health brought me that sense of power that I always felt was lacking. When I took ownership of my health, everything started to get better. I want to empower you to do the same.

In my search for a solution, I realised that my lifestyle was it. While I knew what had healed my skin, and I'd found a system that helped me to stick to the lifestyle changes I'd made, I wasn't clear on why it had worked. And so began a year of research, training in health coaching, facial therapy, anatomy and physiology for therapists, and lots of personal experiments to understand why my skin cleared and how I could sustain the results. I learned how our bodies work and how to treat our skin right. And I realised that changing my habits is what gave me sustainable results.

My skin healed, and it has stayed clear.

On the surface, the changes are quite straightforward. But changing your habits, particularly eating habits, can be hard. You're changing something you've more or less done the same way for much of your life.

I didn't want this book to be a six-week program that left you wondering what to do next, or an unsustainable diet, because let's face it, most diets are unsustainable. I wanted to write a book that helps you to find a way of living life that works for you. To give you the tools that made it easier for me to change so you can do it too.

Once you've read this book, you'll have the knowledge of what to do and a system showing you how to do it, written by someone that's done it and seen results.

I don't claim to be a specialist of any kind. None of the specialists I worked with got me results. I had to figure it all out on my own. To me, it's not about being an expert. It's about contributing to the conversation we need to have about how we better manage acne, eczema, and psoriasis to bring relief to the millions of sufferers around the world. By raising awareness of the effects of skin issues, sharing our stories, and highlighting what's working, more people will find the relief they so desperately need.

PART I

OUR SKIN

1.1 WHAT IS OUR SKIN?

We don't often think of our skin as an organ, but it is. It's the largest organ in our body. It has many essential jobs, including regulating body temperature, keeping pathogens from the environment out, and synthesising vitamin D, which is created in our bodies when our skin is exposed to sunlight.

There are different layers of skin, including:

- **The epidermis** - the waterproof, protective outer layer of skin. The epidermis is comprised of multiple layers, each with its own function. The epidermis continually renews itself. New skin cells are made in the lower layers of the epidermis and move to the top layer within only a few weeks. What you see when you look at your skin is dead skin cells that are being shed on a daily basis.

- **The dermis** – sitting beneath the epidermis is the dermis, where you'll find connective tissue containing collagen and elastin. These fibres make the skin strong yet flexible. It's also home to nerves, sweat glands, oil glands, hair follicles, and blood and lymphatic vessels, transporting nutrients and oxygen to your skin cells and removing waste. The oil glands, also known as sebaceous glands, produce sebum, your skin's natural oil.

- **The subcutaneous layer** – sitting beneath the dermis, the subcutaneous layer anchors the skin to the body. It's made up of fat and connective tissue that insulates and protects your joints, bones, and internal organs. Like the dermis, it also contains glands, nerves, and blood and lymph vessels.

Everyone's skin may have the same job and the same structure, but everyone's skin is different.

My skin might be more sensitive than yours. Mine might react better than yours to particular products or ingredients, and yours might react better than mine to other products or ingredients.

Stop and think about your body for a minute. Could scientists re-create something as sophisticated as the human body?

There's still so much we don't know about how our body works despite the research.

Our bodies have evolved into this incredible life-supporting package that works in ways we're still trying to figure out. It's no wonder there's so little known for sure about acne, eczema, and psoriasis.

Skin conditions may have become more common, but that doesn't mean you just have to live with them. There are things you can do to get some relief. This may include creams and medications, but your lifestyle can also be a key factor in relieving your symptoms.

1.2 WHAT CAUSES SKIN ISSUES?

Did you know that people with psoriasis have an above-average vulnerability to sore throats? In 2012, researchers from Iceland and the USA took 29 psoriasis patients who also suffered from sore throats. They divided them into 2 groups and removed the tonsils from everyone in one of the groups. From the 15 people who had their tonsils removed, 13 saw a long-term improvement in their psoriasis. Those that still had their tonsils reported no improvement.

I read this in the book *Gut* by Guilia Enders. It naturally caught my eye because of my experience with tonsillitis.

Other studies have shown similar results, but no one knows what the connection is other than to say it's likely to be related to the cells of our immune system. Psoriasis is an autoimmune disease, meaning the immune system is either overactive or triggered by something, resulting in problems for the skin. Like acne and eczema, there are different types of psoriasis. The most common form appears as large red and raised patches of skin. Like eczema, the skin is itchy, painful, and can crack and bleed.

For me, was it an infection in my tonsils that led to my immune system overreacting and causing psoriasis? If so, does that also explain why I then went on to develop acne and eczema?

Or was it the many antibiotics I took to fight off tonsillitis causing damage to my gut? That certainly seems to fit given I also developed irritable bowel syndrome. But the truth is, I don't know, and the doctors don't know either.

I mention this study not to encourage you to get your tonsils removed, but rather to show that no one knows what causes skin issues. There are plenty of theories, including:

- A product you're using on your skin
- Other external irritants like cleaning products or products you use at work
- Dust or pet allergens
- A particular food or food group you're eating
- A symptom of stress
- Lack of sleep
- A reaction to medication
- Hormone imbalances
- Inflammation in the body
- An overactive immune system
- Underlying skin infection or medical condition
- Certain medications and antibiotics
- A combination of any of the above

There are lots of theories, and some arguments are certainly more persuasive than others, but there's, as yet, no consensus on a cause for these skin conditions. It's likely a combination of factors that cause them.

Of course, as well as the above possible causes, you've also got people who believe chocolate, sugar, or 'dirty diets' cause skin issues. I would regularly get comments such as "you need to eat less chocolate" and "you should clean up your diet, that'll sort your skin". These comments usually came from people that did not have, and had never had, a problem with their skin. Their view was that I was putting rubbish into my body, so rubbish was coming out of my skin. This view is simplistic and ill-informed in my experience.

How many people do you know that eat a rubbish diet? I know A LOT, and none of them have issues with their skin. Sure, their complexion might be brighter if they ate better, but they do not have acne, eczema, or psoriasis.

When my skin was at its worst, I was acutely aware of my diet. I drank water, tried to eat my five portions of fruit and veg each day, and practised yoga a couple of times a week. My general lifestyle was not unhealthy. Your lifestyle is unlikely to be the cause of your skin condition, but it can be part of your solution.

In this book, I will guide you through an exercise to track back to when your symptoms first appeared. By recalling what was going on in your life, I believe you can find a possible cause for your unique situation. Identifying a likely cause, or at least the lifestyle factors that are exacerbating your skin conditions shows you where to focus your energy most to help you to heal.

1.3 DO YOU HAVE ACNE, ECZEMA, OR PSORIASIS?

I'm not going to cover off what acne, eczema, and psoriasis are. If you have one of these conditions, you already know what it is. You're living with it every day.

What I will say is that it's important not to self-diagnose a skin condition. There are many types of skin conditions. Even within the broad category of chronic skin conditions, there are different types of acne, eczema, and psoriasis.

Some skin conditions will be infinitely more treatable, and a simple box of pills might be just what you need to resolve the issue.

Inflammation on the skin can also be a sign of many other health conditions that need medical treatment.

If your condition has not been formally diagnosed, stop and check-in with your doctor.

1.4 BE KIND TO YOUR SKIN

As well as getting you in the habit of eating well to nourish your skin, I'd like this book to help you change your relationship with your skin.

When you suffer from a skin issue, it's easy to fall into the trap of hating your skin. You get angry and treat it with harsh chemicals to "dry up" spots or weeping sores.

You blame your skin for you not going out, not going swimming, not wearing the same clothes as your friends, not applying for that new job, or whatever else you feel your skin is stopping you from doing.

Your skin doesn't want to be angry and inflamed either. It doesn't want to be scratched until it bleeds. Your skin is sending you a message. It's not trying to ruin your life.

It wants you to look at your lifestyle. Something needs attention, and it's very rarely your skin.

1.5 DO DIET AND LIFESTYLE REALLY IMPACT SKIN?

It affects everything else, so why wouldn't it affect our skin?

Diet directly impacts our blood pressure and our risk of heart disease, cancer, and stroke. A poor diet can lead to type-2 diabetes, and what we eat impacts the health of our bones, our joints, our brain, and the health of our gut.

It seems that every other organ in our body is affected by what we eat, so why wouldn't our skin, which is, remember, the body's largest organ.

Our skin is affected by our emotions. Whatever you're feeling shows up on your skin. If you're embarrassed, your skin goes red. If you feel sick, your skin goes pale. When you're cold, or you feel scared, you get goosebumps. If you're in love, your skin is glowing.

If emotions are reflected so routinely on our skin, it makes sense that whatever is happening within our body can also be reflected on our skin.

Our skin is complex, and there's more we still need to learn.

We might struggle to explain exactly why food affects our skin, but we also struggle to explain exactly how our brain works. There will be things happening inside our bodies that scientists don't even know exist yet.

The world is gradually coming around to accept that diet and lifestyle absolutely affect our skin. What we currently know about our skin and how it's affected by what goes on deep inside of our body is exactly that...what we *currently* know. Give it five or ten years, and science will make a discovery that changes what we think today. Until then, let's look at what we do know.

Why are people not talking about diet and lifestyle when treating skin issues?

People are talking about it. But it's mainly people that have suffered with their skin and found a way of managing their condition through their diet and lifestyle. It's, unfortunately, a discussion that's still not commonplace when seeing doctors and dermatologists.

This has been a big frustration for me over the years. If you look at the organisations supporting skin conditions, it's disappointing that lifestyle factors are rarely mentioned.

Treatment options presented are usually restricted to what you might call conventional treatments, including products applied directly to the skin such as topical steroids and emollients, antibiotics, oral steroids, retinoid and immuno-suppressant drugs, ultraviolet light therapy, and the contra-ceptive pill.

If I can put my conspiracy theorist hat on for just a second, these are all treatments that are made by pharmaceutical companies. They will work to varying degrees, but some of these treatments require a lifetime of medication. Many have side effects, and most will fail to deliver long term. Money is not spent analysing the effect of lifestyle factors on skin conditions because no one will make money from it.

We're no longer reliant solely on the information our doctor and pharmaceutical companies give us. We can see and hear from real people who have had real results. There are countless ways people are sharing their personal stories of what's worked and what hasn't for their skin.

The medical community is also changing. We're seeing doctors stepping outside of their traditional role and advocating lifestyle changes. They're writing books, blogs, and podcasts to tell us lifestyle does matter, and for some health conditions, it's more effective than any pill could ever be.

We're also seeing a real shift in our use of, and attitude towards, antibiotics. There are now posters up in my local GP surgery and my pharmacy window saying that antibiotics will not treat your common cold, and taking them when you don't really need them puts you and your family at risk.

It's also much more widely known that antibiotics kill the bacteria in our gut, good and bad, making our microbiome much less diverse. We're going to look at why this is relevant to your skin shortly.

What's not clear is how long it takes the gut to recover from a course of antibiotics. Some studies suggest that certain species of microbes recover within just a few weeks following antibiotics. In contrast, other species can remain depleted for many months, if not indefinitely, and the long-term effects of this are not known.

I don't write this to knock antibiotics. It's just a fact. We should take antibiotics when we need them. The knowledge we now have of what effect they have inside our bodies means we're better able to minimise any unintended consequences by taking probiotics and feeding our gut the types of foods necessary to replenish our gut bacteria.

I've had to take antibiotics since healing my skin. With each prescription, I've asked if it's a good idea to take probiotics too. With each question, I was told yes, it is a good idea. It's disappointing that this information was never volunteered; I've had to ask every time, but it's still a good sign.

As a trained health coach, I see the value in the medical community working in partnership with those advocating lifestyle changes. Diseases such as heart attacks, strokes, cancer, and diabetes kill 41 million people every year. This is equivalent to 71% of deaths globally, according to the World Health Organisation's 2018 factsheet on noncommunicable diseases.

The World Health Organisation lists behavioural factors including physical inactivity, unhealthy diet, tobacco use, and the harmful use of alcohol, combined with genetic and environmental factors, as the key risk factors behind the development of these diseases.

We're slowly opening our eyes to other ways of managing some common health conditions. The more people talk about the amazing benefits they're experiencing by changing their lifestyle, the more others will be inspired to change theirs.

The medication you choose to take is a decision for you. What's right for one might not be what's right for another. I don't think medication is a bad thing. Sometimes we all need to take it. But if that medication is just a sticking plaster to help you to manage the symptoms of your skin issues, your lifestyle might be the thing that brings you longer-term relief.

If you are taking medication, it's always a good idea to ask your doctor if they're aware of any steps you can take to minimise potential side effects.

Whichever path you take, optimising your diet and lifestyle for great health is always a good thing to do.

PART II

A HEALTHY DIET

2.1 WHAT IS A HEALTHY DIET?

Most people would like to eat a healthier diet but are put off by various obstacles that get in their way.

Does any of this sound familiar? You're too busy, or you don't know how to cook. It's too expensive to buy healthy food. You've tried to eat a healthier diet, but your family won't eat it, and you don't want to have to cook two different meals.

Or perhaps you're struggling because you don't know what a healthy diet is.

With so many different diets, theories, conflicting advice, and changing viewpoints, it can get overwhelming. What's good for you one month is bad for you the next and vice versa.

Despite all of this noise, what I see in every diet is:

1. eating fruits and vegetables, and
2. drinking water is good for you.

These two principles, to me, are the foundations of a healthy diet. They're what I added into my daily routine, and they're the focus of this book.

It took me a long time and lots of trial and error to find something that relieved my symptoms. And when I found it, I realised just how simple it was.

Removing foods was never going to work because I was missing the proper foundations of healthy eating. It's like building a house. If you don't lay the right foundations, your house will crumble. But get those foundations right, and you've got yourself a stable home for years to come.

I'm not an expert in food nutrition. I don't know how much vitamin C is in an orange or the recommended daily intake of protein. I don't need to know this, and I don't think you need to either.

The nutritional benefits of the food we're eating are not something we think about every day. And while that might well be part of the problem, that's not going to change. We're all too busy to make sure our meals have the right ratio of protein, fat, and healthy carbs. In any case, the "right ratio" and "what constitutes a healthy carb" are often hotly debated.

What we can do, and with much greater ease, is make sure we're eating plenty of fruit and vegetables — a simple, non-controversial health goal, universally acknowledged as a healthy habit.

Let's look at why we should eat more fruit and vegetables. Truly understanding why is a good way of reframing it in your mind so you actually do it.

Why should we care about eating fruit and vegetables?

Have you noticed everyone is talking about gut health? That's because scientists and the medical profession have figured out your gut is one your body's most critical organs. It significantly influences your physical health, your mental health, and your risk of developing future diseases.

According to the World Health Organisation, people whose diets are rich in vegetables and fruit have a significantly lower risk of obesity, heart disease, stroke, diabetes, and certain types of cancer.

It's believed this lower risk is due to our gut bacteria. A gut health book I highly recommend is *Gut Reactions* by Justin and Erica Sonnenburg. The book argues that the richness (or lack of richness) of your microbiome is a better predictor of Western disease risk than your weight. Those with a richer microbiome eat a wider variety of fruit and vegetables than those with a poorer microbiome.

While there's undoubtedly more to come from research on the gut, what we know so far is our bodies are one big ecosystem with trillions of bacteria living on and in them, a significant amount of which live in our gut. Some of these bacteria, collectively known as our microbiome, are friendly, and some are not.

Those little microbes in your gut are fundamental to your overall health and wellbeing. Each species seems to thrive off different sources of dietary fibre. We get dietary fibre from eating plants, including fruit, vegetables, legumes, and certain grains.

Eating a wide variety of fruit and vegetables gives us the best chance of achieving a harmonious balance of gut bacteria to keep us in the best health. Basically, the good bugs love fruit and veg, so we want to feed them well.

I like to think of my gut as being like the Trolls movie. Stay with me for a minute here! When you can see a picture rather than an abstract concept, it is much easier to connect with why you are doing something.

Try visualising this little world inside your gut as a community of microbes waiting for their next meal. When you feed them well with lots of fruits and vegetables, it's like party time for the Trolls. There are bright colours, blooming flowers, music, dancing, and happy faces everywhere.

But when you're not eating what your microbes need, your gut morphs into Bergen Town. A dark, dreary place where the inhabitants trudge around singing the song "I ain't happy". Google the song if you've not seen the film.

Visualising what's going on inside you is also a great way of getting children to eat their veggies. If you have kids, sit them down and talk to them about their microbes, or gut bugs, as we call them in my house. Explain that they have little pets (or Trolls) inside them, and it's their job to look after them. Giving children a reason that's more than 'because it's good for you' gets them to rethink why you're making them eat their veggies.

2.2 THE GUT SKIN CONNECTION

If you're wondering why I'm talking about gut health in a book about skin, it's because of the gut skin connection that I touched on earlier. There is an increasing number of scientific studies linking our skin's health to the health of our gut.

Two conditions of the gut, in particular, have been linked to skin conditions.

Gut dysbiosis is when there's an imbalance between the friendly and unfriendly microbes in the gut; and leaky gut, which is where your gut lining is compromised, allowing undigested particles of food to leak through to your bloodstream.

Both of these gut conditions are thought to have the potential to impact skin function and trigger a reaction from your immune system contributing to several health conditions, including acne, eczema, and psoriasis.

Research into gut health is still new, but the scientific studies combined with the results people see when they take action to improve their gut health are promising.

The very existence of leaky gut has been subject to much debate in the medical and scientific communities. If you're a gut health sceptic, I encourage you to read the book *The Clever Guts Diet*. The author, Dr Michael Mosley, is open about his scepticism in the past but writes that there is now clear evidence that leaky gut is a real condition, occurring for many reasons including a gut infection, poor diet, or the use of antibiotics.

These debates demonstrate just part of the issue with our gut health. It's difficult to confirm something as fact. Our gut has been neglected for many years, perhaps understandably given it's not the sexiest part of the body to study. The good news is we're beginning to recognise there's another world that we don't know much about living right inside each of us. The more research that's carried out into this world, the greater the chance we can positively impact many health conditions, including acne, eczema, and psoriasis.

With the benefit of hindsight and the emerging studies on gut health, I can see what happened with my skin. It wasn't a coincidence that my skin issues developed at the same time as recurring tonsillitis, antibiotics every month for a year and a half, and irritable bowel syndrome. My gut was not in a good state, and this was reflected on my skin.

Around 70% of our immune system is in our gut. Psoriasis is an autoimmune disease, meaning the immune system is either overactive or triggered by something. I don't think it's too much of a stretch to suggest that an unhappy and perhaps leaky gut could well have triggered my psoriasis.

It also wasn't a coincidence that the more fruits and vegetables I ate, the better my skin got. The new colour and variety in my diet improved my gut health by giving the friendly bacteria what they need to multiply and thrive. Improving my gut health gave my body what it needed to heal my skin.

Jeanette Hyde summarises it nicely in her book *The Gut Makeover* when she says to have beautiful skin, we need to support our microbiome. This was certainly my experience and is why this book is so focused on getting you in the habit of eating in a way that supports a healthy gut.

Can't I just take a probiotic to sort my gut out?

No. Just like you can't supplement your way out of an unhealthy diet, you can't supplement your way into a healthy gut. Though there certainly is a place for probiotics.

I was on holiday in France and myself and a number of the other hotel guests came down with a bout of food poisoning. From speaking with some of the other guests, everyone that had the salmon for dinner was now ill. Thankfully, this experience didn't put me off salmon, which is excellent for skin health.

I went to the local pharmacy and asked for something to make me feel a bit better. The pharmacist thankfully spoke English because my French was terrible. He gave me three boxes of pills.

The first box would help to reduce nausea. The second box was an antibiotic to kill the bacteria causing the food poisoning. The third box was a probiotic.

The pharmacist explained that the antibiotic would kill the bugs in my system, good and bad, and the probiotic would help replenish the good bugs caught in the antibiotic crossfire.

Probiotics are live bacteria. You can take probiotics to repopulate your gut with friendly bacteria, so they help if your gut is not in great shape or you've been taking antibiotics.

I do take a probiotic at various points throughout the year. If you are going to take probiotics, shop around. Different brands contain different strains of probiotics, and scientists don't yet know which strains are most effective for which health condition. You can take a probiotic, but you won't know if you're getting the most effective strain to help your skin.

Try a few different types and see if you notice a difference. I use the multi-strain biotic from Wild Nutrition. When I take it, I notice a difference, and that's what I'm after. But your microbiome is different from mine, so you might need to try different probiotics to feel the benefits.

That said, your body will always benefit more from feeding it the way nature intended rather than relying on something made in a lab. And besides, once you've swallowed down a bunch of new microbes, you still need to feed them.

Probiotic foods

You can also top up your friendly bacteria by including the following foods in your diet.

- Cheese that contains live cultures
- Fermented sauerkraut and other pickled vegetables
- Fermented miso paste
- Kefir and live yogurt
- Kimchi
- Kombucha

To get the benefit of the live bacteria, these products should be stored in the fridge. You're looking for the fermented products rather than the pasteurised type that's shelf-stable.

Prebiotic foods

Prebiotics provide food for your microbes and help them do a better job of supporting your digestive system. You can find prebiotics in the following foods.

- Apples
- Asparagus
- Bananas
- Chicory
- Flaxseeds
- Garlic
- Leeks
- Oats
- Onions
- Pak Choi
- Potatoes, served cooked but cold

I list these foods here for interest only. The best way to make sure you're eating well is to focus on eating a wide variety of fruits and vegetables. Don't limit yourself to only a handful of different vegetables, even if they are considered to be prebiotic.

You don't need to be a vegetarian to eat vegetables

Before we look at the habits, let's get one thing out of the way for those worried I'm trying to turn you veggie. You don't need to be a vegetarian to eat vegetables.

There's been an explosion of vegetarian and vegan options recently. With some people arguing less meat is better for your health, others arguing it's better for the environment.

Hard-core viewpoints from veggies and meat-eaters alike are everywhere.

My view is you don't need to pick a side. You can eat meat and eat a lot of vegetables. It doesn't need to be an either-or.

I was a vegetarian for six years, and I was unhealthy. My doctor told me my vegetarian diet wasn't right for me and advised me to start eating meat again. I took his advice and went back to eating meat. Guess what happened? Nothing. I was still unhealthy.

I know now I wasn't unhealthy because of a lack of meat. I was unhealthy because my diet was lacking variety. I didn't eat enough fruit and vegetables, and my gut was in a pretty sorry state.

Regardless of your philosophical views of meat, eating vegetables is good for you, so just do it whether or not you also eat meat.

PART III

GETTING STARTED

3.1 GETTING STARTED

Right, this is the chapter where I put you to work.

Hopefully, you've come to realise that there's not one thing that's going to heal your skin. It's a collection of things done repeatedly that will make the difference.

In the same way one session in the gym will not transform your abs, one skin treatment, or one healthy meal, or one day of managing your stress will not transform your skin. But being kind to your skin and looking after your body inside and out repeatedly will. It's going to take a lifetime of eating well to heal then maintain your new healthy body and skin.

The nine habits of eating well in this book are not that hard. But they do require you to change a set of habits you've done the same way for much of your life, your eating habits.

The way we eat is called our eating habits because we eat pretty much the same foods, at the same time, in the same places, with the same people, and in the same way for years.

But the great thing about building healthy habits is that we are creatures of habit. Once we've made something a habit, we'll do it automatically and reap the benefits for life without even thinking about it.

It ceases to be hard. It just becomes the way we do things.

In a minute, I'm going to ask you to reflect on your skin story. Doing this is a great way to flag up possible causes or triggers for your acne, eczema, or psoriasis.

We're then going to look at the nine habits.

We'll finish by looking at the strategies and techniques you can use to implement them because knowing something isn't enough. It's doing something with that knowledge that gets results.

But first, I'm going to cover off a question I get asked a lot.

3.2 SHOULD I CONSULT MY DOCTOR?

Yes. This book offers no medical advice. It's a book about how changing my eating habits helped to heal my skin with information on how you can do the same. But anyone embarking on a change of diet and lifestyle should consult their doctor in the first instance.

We're fortunate that we live in a time where there's more awareness than ever before about health conditions. There's also more information than there has ever been before. This can sometimes be overwhelming. We get stuck in a state of research and never put anything into action. Or we get sucked down the path of natural healing and turn away from anything that our doctor may tell us.

Like vegetables and meat, you can have the best of both worlds.

You can change your lifestyle to heal your body and skin, and you can use the medication your doctor prescribes to help you to manage the symptoms. No one says you can't try both.

If you're taking medication in the form of antibiotics or immunosuppressant's, talk to your doctor about how best to minimise the side effects and tell them you want to look at your lifestyle too.

My view is to take all the help you can get from conventional medicine to help bring you temporary relief. But alongside this, do what you can to take good care of your gut microbes, and they'll be able to do a better job of taking care of you.

3.3 GETTING STARTED EXERCISES

I'm going to ask you to reflect on what else was going on in your life at the time your skin issues started. I've seen people realise stress triggers their skin issues given they first appeared alongside a major life event, exams or key times of stress at work. I've seen others realise it's the products they're using on their skin or the chemicals they are exposed to every day in their workplace.

While the best way to manage skin issues is a healthy balance of lifestyle factors, this exercise can help you to see which areas of your lifestyle you should pay particular attention to.

Grab your phone, a notepad and a pen and complete the following exercises.

1. Skin story – part one

In your notebook, write down your skin story. Use the following questions to help you.

- How old were you when your skin issues first started?
- What was going on in your life at that time?
- What significant changes happened?
- What job were you doing?
- What other health concerns did you have at the time?
- What medication were you taking?
- What was your typical diet?
- What was your typical exercise routine?
- How stressed did you feel?
- Did you have any issues sleeping?

2. Skin story – part two

Now think of your most significant flare-up.

Use the same questions plus any others you've thought of, but thinking about your lifestyle at the time of that flare-up.

3. Take photos of your skin.

My skin was at its worst before the days of selfies thankfully, but I encourage you to take photos. You don't have to show them to anyone but taking photos is a great way to help you to see the progress you're making. It isn't easy when you see your skin every day to see improvements but looking back in one month, three months, or six months can show you what you've achieved.

4. Write down where on your body your acne, eczema, or psoriasis is.

Keeping note of this is another great way to keep track of your progress. When you look back at your notes, you might realise you've forgotten all about that patch of eczema you used to have on your wrist, for example.

5. Write down all of your symptoms.

And I mean ALL of your symptoms. Start at your head and make your way down to your toes, taking note of all symptoms. When my skin healed, my irritable bowel syndrome was better. But I also realised that my headaches were gone, I couldn't remember the last time I had heartburn, my recurring sinusitis and constant stuffy nose were a thing of the past. We tend not to think of some of these little niggling health conditions as symptoms. They're just things everyone experiences. But just because lots of people have them doesn't mean they're normal. They're a sign that something is wrong. You'll be amazed at how many of these common health conditions clear up when you change your eating habits.

6. Track your energy levels.

How tired to do you feel on a scale of 1–10? What you eat directly contributes to how much energy you have. This is not just another measurement of your progress. Being more aware of your energy levels will help you further down the line to identify the foods that make you feel healthy and energised and the foods that make you feel sluggish and tired.

7. Get the all-clear from your doctor.

It's a good idea to discuss any insights you've had with your doctor plus get the all-clear from your doctor before you start making changes to your lifestyle.

Getting Started Key Steps

1. Write down your skin story – part one.
2. Write down your skin story – part two.
3. Take photos of your skin.
4. Note where on your body your skin issues are.
5. Write down ALL of your symptoms, starting with your head and working your way down to your toes.
6. Track your energy levels on a scale of 1–10.
7. Get the all-clear from your doctor.

Remember that this book will work for you if you do the work, so please do these exercises.

If you've done them, great, you're ready to go. Join me in the next chapter where we'll dive into your new eating habits.

PART IV

EATING HABITS FOR HEALTHY SKIN

4.1 HABIT 1 – FALL IN LOVE WITH FOOD AGAIN

Let's start by talking about our relationship with food, and some of the anxiety associated with it. Please note that I'm not talking about eating disorders here. If you have a history of disordered eating, then this is not the book for you. Put it down and speak with an appropriate healthcare professional.

Whenever I tried to change my diet in the past, I found it so difficult and unsustainable. I always felt restricted, like I was on a diet, and I had a big list of foods I couldn't eat. Everything I ate needed planning and special ingredients shopped for or ordered online. Every meal felt difficult.

This was because everything I tried meant removing lots of foods from my diet. There might be foods you find out you need to limit or exclude, but chances are it's just one or two things. Your list of what you eat should be WAY bigger than any list of what you don't eat.

Skin issues aside, food has somehow become one of the most contentious subjects out there.

I look at my daughter and food, for her, is something she eats when she's hungry. Once she's eaten her food, she bounces up from the table and gets on with her day. She just eats and goes. She knows that her meals are healthy, and she knows that apples are healthier snacks than sweeties. Most of the time she'll have the apple, sometimes she'll have the sweeties. She doesn't overthink it. She doesn't feel guilty about her food choices.

I don't know how old we are when this changes, or even why it changes. But it does change. Along the way, we lose sight of what food is. We associate food with feelings of guilt, we judge ourselves for our food choices, and we judge others for theirs.

Everyone has an opinion on what we should and shouldn't be eating. And when someone finds a style of eating that works for them, they often become evangelical about it.

Foods get labelled as good and bad, and the labels change depending on who you are talking to and what their eating habits are. When we make changes to our diet, we can get accused of going on a faddy diet, which to be fair, sometimes we are.

We post photos of our breakfast, lunch and dinner online, which isn't necessarily a bad thing. I now eat more avocados in a month than I ate in the first 30 years of my life.

But when you have an issue with your skin, all of this can be stressful. You think people are judging you for eating chocolate or chips. If you're eliminating lots of foods, you don't want to go out to that party because there won't be anything there you can eat, or you don't want to seem fussy by asking the waitress to leave certain ingredients off your plate. Food can easily become the cause of social anxiety and isolation.

I don't claim to be able to solve any of this. But when food becomes part of a healing journey, as it did for me, that fact alone changes your relationship with food all over again.

I encourage you to look at your food choices slightly differently. To see that what you eat matters more than what you don't eat.

When I shifted my mindset from cutting food out to adding lots of goodness in, I saw food for what it is; nourishment for my body as well as a bit of nourishment for my soul... chocolate, I'm looking at you.

Learning more about what's going on inside my body also helped me to change my mindset around food. The nourishment my gut needs now influences the food I put on my plate every day.

Make good food memories

Another way to fall in love with food again is to make good food memories.

In 2011, I went to Vietnam with my husband. We took the train from Ho Chi Minh City to Hanoi, a 35-hour journey. We boarded the train early in the morning. It was still dark and too early for breakfast in our hotel. We jumped aboard, planning to buy some breakfast on the train. We found our cabin, a tiny room with four narrow beds, two up and two down. We settled in and said hello to our Vietnamese roommates.

Once the train had pulled away from the station and our

journey was underway, my husband went off in search of food. He returned after only a few minutes and said there was no food cart on the train. I've always loved breakfast, so this was a blow! Instead of eating, we watched the Vietnamese countryside go by from the small window in our cabin. We thought there must be some provisions for food on-board given the journey was all day and all night.

Sure enough, at lunchtime, a lady appeared in the corridor outside our cabin with a pan of food. We took a look in the pan. It was some kind of dark soup. We decided against it, hoping that another trolley would come along.

About 8 pm, the same lady appeared with her trolley. She looked at us and raised her eyebrows. We nodded. Whatever was on the menu for dinner, we were having it. We were famished.

The lady spooned rice into take-out containers then picked up meat patties. She chopped them up with rusty looking scissors, picked up a plastic bottle and squirted a dark, watery sauce over each meal before handing them to us.

The now sliced pattie looked like meat, tasted like fish and, to this day, I have no idea what it was we ate. But it was one of the tastiest meals we've ever had and one of my favourite memories from Vietnam.

My point is how many of our favourite memories have food in them? We celebrate with food. Whether it's birthday parties, Christmas or weddings, we remember the food because it means something to us.

Go out of your way to make some new good food memories. When you're celebrating something, choose restaurants or recipes you wouldn't usually to make it just that little bit extra special.

When you're on holiday, seek out restaurants frequented by locals. You'll find the food is authentic, tastier, and cheaper than the typical tourist restaurants. Try recreating some of your favourite meals when you get home.

Quick tips for loving your food now

If that anniversary dinner or summer holiday is still a way off for you, here are some quick tips you can do today to make your meals more satisfying and encourage a more positive relationship with food:

- Focus on your food. How many times have you eaten at your desk or in front of the TV and you can't remember your meal? For me, too many times to count. Eat at your kitchen table if you have one. Minimise distractions by taking yourself away from your desk at work, or at least shut your emails off so you can pay more attention to your food, which brings me neatly on to my next suggestion.

- Savour your food. Use all of your senses and notice the flavours, the sight, the smell. This has the added benefit of being good for your digestion. Your digestive juices start flowing once your eyes register a tasty meal in front of you. Stop eating on auto-pilot, and you'll quickly remember how good it is to enjoy your food.

- Enjoy the social side of eating. Sit at the table, eat as

a family or make a commitment to eat with a friend every week. Make mealtimes something you look forward to. You don't need to do this every day if you're all on different schedules. But eat together whenever you can, even if that's only one or two days at the weekend. If you have children, you'll find they're much more willing to try new foods if they see others in the family enjoying them too.

- Enjoy your eating environment. Light a candle, use beautiful plates and play relaxing music in the background. There's something about beautiful crockery that makes you treat it better. You want to fill it with vibrant food, which means more of the good stuff.

- I love eating from bowls. There's been an explosion of recipes online and even full recipe books dedicated to 'bowl food'. I don't know where this came from, but I love it. Bowls have the hygge-effect. They somehow make the food so much more comforting, as though you're curled up on the sofa under a blanket.

- If you eat lunch at work, get fancy packed lunch boxes. I like the ones with lots of little compartments. Most of what you prepare at home is going to be far better for you than what you can grab from your work canteen or local coffee shop. My daughter loves those insulated bowls. I put hot food in it in the morning and it's still warm for her at lunchtime.

- Make a conscious effort to become a foodie. Enjoy trying new foods. You won't like them all, but you will find some dishes you love, which will make eating a more varied diet easier for you.

Actions:

- Shift your mindset from cutting foods out to adding goodness in. Stop associating food with negative emotions. Instead, start viewing food as nourishment.

- Enjoy your food, savour every mouthful and go out of your way to make new food memories.

4.2 HABIT 2 – BANISH THE BEIGE

Many of the staples in our diet are beige. Whether you're eating toast, porridge, cereal, sandwiches, pasta, rice, or potatoes, they are all somewhat lacking in colour.

Bringing awareness to the colour, or lack of, on your plate makes you think differently about it. When you think differently, you behave differently.

Whenever I serve a meal, be it breakfast, lunch, or dinner, I think of the phrase Banish the Beige and look for ways to add colour to my plate. By doing this, I naturally eat a lot more fruit and vegetables than I ever did before.

It's so easy. I no longer need to think about it. I automatically add handfuls of fruit, vegetables, nuts, and seeds to every meal.

Prepare your food as you usually would then look at how you can brighten it up.

Here are two easy ways to get started:

1. Add some greens

Leafy greens give you the biggest bang for your buck when you first start eating more veg. Greens are packed full of vitamins, minerals, antioxidants, and fibre. They should be in a category all of their own because they're such nutrient powerhouses.

Darker leafy greens typically contain more nutrients than their paler counterparts. Introduce spinach, kale, rocket, and chard into your diet. They're widely available and easy to prepare and cook. They can also be eaten raw in a salad or smoothie.

Here are some ideas to help you easily integrate more leafy greens into your daily routine:

- Pak Choi – slice it up and add it to stir-fries, soups, and omelettes
- Spinach – add a handful to smoothies, omelettes, pasta dishes, sandwiches and salads
- Kale – stir-fry it in coconut oil and freshly sliced chilli, add to curry dishes
- Rocket – add to salads, on the side of scrambled eggs, as a topping for pasta or pizza
- Chard – slice and add to smoothies

The more you eat, the better they taste, so get chomping.

Action:

Buy a bag of greens in your food shop this week and eat them. If you prefer to drink your greens, you'll find green smoothie recipes at www.thelifestylecircle.com.

2. Add all of the other colours too

Adding lots of different colours is an easy way to eat a variety of different fruit and vegetables.

Richly coloured plants are high in polyphenols, says Jeanette Hyde, Nutritional Therapist and author of *The Gut Makeover*. These polyphenols are the plant chemicals that give plants their colour. They're also a rich source of food for our gut microbes and the cause of the health transformations Jeanette sees with her clients.

A helpful variation of Banish the Beige is making LOADED your new favourite word.

When I hear loaded I think of loaded potato skins. Where the cooked inside of the potato is scooped out, mixed with other ingredients, and then stuffed back into the potato skin.

Loaded is a useful word because, alongside Banish the Beige, it reminds me to load my dish with as many different fruit and vegetables as I can. Loaded meals are everyday meals loaded with extra goodness.

You can use the principles of Banish the Beige and Loaded interchangeably or pick the one that resonates most with you.

Examples of LOADED meals

Loaded Breakfasts

- Scrambled eggs with spinach, tomatoes and chives topped with a sprinkling of pumpkin seeds.

- Porridge with cinnamon, chia seeds, grated apple, and a handful of raisins.

- Sourdough toast topped with spinach, mashed avocado, and baked tomatoes.

- Granola topped with extra pumpkin seeds, coconut flakes, juicy cranberries, flaked almonds, and fresh banana slices.

- Omelette with cheese and ham plus onion, peppers, tomatoes, chives, and a handful of fresh rocket.

Loaded Lunches

- Ham sandwiches made from fresh baguette with good quality ham, pickled gherkin, and spinach.

- Cheese sandwiches with sourdough bread. Vary your cheese and your fillings. Lettuce, tomatoes, red onion, peppers, green chilli, or pickles work well.

- Hummus wraps with hummus, roasted courgette, peppers, onions, and fresh rocket.

- Tuna mayo sandwiches with sourdough bread and tuna, mayonnaise, celery, and red onion.

- Grilled cheese with ciabatta bread, and topped with sautéed mushrooms, onions, tomatoes, and spinach. Cover with shredded cheese and grill until the cheese melts.

- Baked potato with cheese, spring onions, sautéed tomatoes, peppers, mushrooms, and kale.

Loaded salads

- Anything goes in a salad so think wider than lettuce, cucumber, and tomatoes.

- Experiment with mixed leafy greens and try your vegetables raw, roasted, sautéed, or steamed.

- Go for a combination of vegetables, seeds, and beans. Any supermarket will have a wide range of healthy salad ingredients, such as sundried tomatoes, peppers, courgettes, onions, sweet corn, peas, edamame beans, beetroot, radishes, carrots, chickpeas, butter beans, avocado, pumpkin seeds, sunflower seeds, sesame seeds, dried cranberries, broccoli, green beans, pickled vegetables, or sauerkraut.

- You can bulk out a salad with rice, pasta, noodles, potatoes, feta cheese, goats cheese, mozzarella, smoked salmon, baked salmon, tuna, mackerel, chicken, eggs, quiche, frittata, or falafel.

- You can make easy salad dressings from lemon or lime juice, and olive oil. Add pressed garlic, any herbs and spices, or mustard for an extra flavour hit. Or keep it simple and add a spoon of hummus or pesto.

- You can also stir-fry many of the above ingredients for a quick and nutritious dinner.

Loaded Dinners

- Pasta dishes, like salads, are wonderfully versatile. Almost anything goes with pasta, so go beyond pesto, cheese, and Bolognese. Use a combination of any of the ingredients in the loaded salad above. Make loaded pasta once a week to use up whatever vegetables are left in the fridge before your next food shop.

- Even macaroni cheese can become loaded if you add mushrooms, onions, tomatoes, and peas. If you're a mac 'n' cheese purist and don't want to mess with the classic recipe, serve it with a big green salad.

- A stir-fry is quick, easy, and nutritious. Use a combination of any of the ingredients in the loaded salad above. Like pasta, a stir-fry once a week is a great way of using up leftovers.

- Chilli is another everyday meal that's easy to spruce up. Prepare your chilli as you normally would with onions, chilli and kidney beans but add a few other ingredients such as black beans, fresh tomatoes, red pepper, yellow pepper, grated carrot, grated courgette, peas, or spinach. For even more goodness, serve your chilli with fresh guacamole made from mashed avocado, tomatoes, lime juice, and a fresh herb such as coriander or parsley.

- Curry is another dish where almost anything goes. You can add onions, chickpeas, sweet potato, spinach, kale, peas, tomatoes, peppers, courgette, green beans, baby corn, broccoli, cauliflower, mange tout, sugar snap peas, pak choi, and fresh herbs.

- Top your burger with lettuce, chopped onions, pickled gherkins, sliced tomato, and roasted peppers. Serve with a big green salad and a combination of sweet potato and regular fries.

The possibilities are endless. These are just some examples to show you how easy it can be to add one or two extra varieties or fruit or vegetables to your favourite meals.

Whether you cook your meals from scratch or use jar and packet sauces, you can still get the gut and skin health benefits by taking an extra couple of minutes to add fresh, healthy ingredients.

Action:

Eat what you usually eat but make a conscious effort to add colour to your meals this week.

Grab your phone and set a reminder to Banish the Beige. Most of us eat at the same time every day. It's easy to pop a reminder into your phone before your usual breakfast, lunch, or dinner time.

A word of caution, if you're not used to eating much fibre, which, given you're reading this book, you're probably not, make the changes gradually. A sudden increase in fibre can make you temporarily gassy.

You may find cooked vegetables easier on your digestive system than raw in the beginning.

4.3 HABIT 3 – EAT 20 - 30 DIFFERENT FRUITS AND VEGETABLES EACH WEEK

With fruit and vegetables, variety is essential. Remember that your gut microbes thrive when you eat a wide range of fruit and vegetables.

Dr. Michael Mosley, in his book *The Clever Guts Diet*, recommends aiming to eat 20 – 30 different varieties of fruit and vegetables every week.

At first glance, this can seem like a lot, but it's surprisingly easy once you get going. Use habit 2 – Banish the Beige - to get you started.

You might eat a bowl of porridge for breakfast, a sandwich for lunch, and pasta for dinner. If you Banish the Beige, these meals might look like this:

- Breakfast - porridge with cinnamon, raisins, and grated apple.

- Lunch - a sandwich with sourdough bread,

hummus, rocket, roasted red and yellow peppers, and sliced red onion.

- Dinner - pasta with spring onions, garlic, fresh tomatoes, peas, chopped spinach, and a handful of fresh parsley.

- Snacks – a banana, sliced nectarine with yogurt, flaked almonds, and pumpkin seeds, and a chocolate bar.

You've just eaten **14 different varieties** of fruit and vegetables in one day plus fresh herbs, spices, nuts, and seeds. And you've done it with meals that are familiar to you and quick and easy to prepare.

UK health advice is to eat 5 portions of fruit and vegetables a day. It's a specific and measurable goal. It's often heralded as a success because it's so well-known. But I don't think it's working for us anymore because people are just not doing it.

There are many suggested reasons for this, one of which is confusion over how many grams of green beans you need to eat or how many cherry tomatoes make one portion.

When you focus on getting 20 – 30 different varieties of fruit and vegetables, you can forget about portion sizes. It doesn't matter if you ate 60g or 80g of green beans. The goal is to eat green beans.

Action:

Go to www.thelifestylecircle.com/bookbonuses and print off the fruit and veg tracker.

Put it somewhere convenient where you'll see it every day. Then start using it.

Get your family engaged with this one. It's incredible how a little bit of competition helps everyone to eat that bit more veg.

4.4 HABIT 4 – FOLLOW THE 80/20 PRINCIPLE

Habit 4 is follow the 80/20 principle, which means eat delicious, healthy food most of the time and a bit of whatever else you fancy some of the time. There's nothing new in this advice, but so many of us struggle to follow it because of our habits.

One of my favourite quotes is from Gretchen Rubin in her book *Better than Before*. Gretchen says, "what we do every day matters more than what we do once in a while".

This is such a powerful philosophy for healthy eating. There isn't any need for an all or nothing approach to diet.

We're often faced with people saying you need to be gluten-free, dairy-free, sugar-free, vegetarian, vegan, or whatever other labels you can think of.

While I'm not against any of these eating styles if they're working for the individual, I think most of us need a bit more flexibility around our eating habits. It's hard these days to stick to a diet that's all of the good stuff, and, as we talked about earlier, there's a lot of debate about what the good stuff is.

The 80/20 principle is a well-known principle. You may have heard it called Pareto's Principle, named after the 19th century economist who first observed it. It's been used to show everything from 80% of results coming from 20% of effort to 20% of your clothes being worn 80% of the time.

I use the 80/20 principle to remind you not to get obsessive about eating well 100% of the time.

There's no point in telling yourself you'll never eat chocolate or drink gin again. If you set yourself these lifetime restrictions, the only thing you'll do is fail. It's just not realistic for the vast majority of people.

Consistency is key. In the same way walking 20 minutes every day is far better for you than running a marathon once in your life, eating well 80% of the time is far better for you than eating well 100% of the time for a week then gorging on junk food for the following week.

Choose to nourish yourself from the inside out and make that choice consistently.

How to apply the 80/20 principle to eating well

- Free yourself from feeling guilty about the food you eat. Accept that not everything in your diet is going to be good for you. Most of your food choices will be. Some won't be, and that's OK.

- Use the 80/20 principle to plan your food. If you

know you're going out for a three-course meal in the evening, choose that day to have a green smoothie for breakfast and a loaded salad for lunch. It'll stop you from overeating, and you'll enjoy your dinner so much more because you won't be stuffed from a carb-heavy lunch.

- Healthy follows Unhealthy. Plan a healthier meal on either side of an unhealthy one and you can have your takeaway *and* stay on track with your new habits. Don't let one unhealthy meal become three unhealthy meals and two unhealthy snacks. It's easy to have one unhealthy meal, think you've ruined the whole day, and binge on rubbish for the rest of the day. Use Healthy follows Unhealthy to give yourself permission to eat that takeaway with a clear next step so your emotions don't get the better of you leading to a weekend eating binge.

- Stop focusing on all the 'bad' things you ate in the day. I see people who get so frustrated with themselves because they ate a cookie or a chocolate bar. They kick themselves for what they perceive to be a failure. But the reality is often somewhat different. Ask them to tell you what else they ate that day and you'll find they've had apples, bananas, spinach, onions, carrots, asparagus, green beans, or whatever else they've added to their meals. Keep your food choices in perspective. You haven't failed because you've had one bar of chocolate. The chocolate was simply part of your 20%. Congratulate yourself for all of the nutritious food you've eaten in the day.

The importance of balance

In the same way it's possible to obsess over chocolate, it's possible to obsess over healthy eating.

Progress, not perfection, is the aim.

You're not aiming for a diet that is 100% the good stuff. You can do that IF (note the big IF) that's the type of thing that lights you up or if you don't like cake, chips or chocolate. But if you're doing it because you feel you have to, or someone will judge you if you don't, then that's not a healthy place to be.

Aiming for the good old 80/20 principle is my healthy place. 80% of the time, I eat well, move my body, manage my stress and take care of my skin on the outside, and 20% of the time, I drink chai lattes, eat chocolate buttons, and binge-watch Queer Eye.

80/20 is a good principle for life in general.

Action:

Give yourself permission now to use the 80/20 principle in your diet and lifestyle.

4.5 HABIT 5 - KEEP AN EYE ON THE COLOUR OF YOUR PEE

This habit is all about drinking more water. Before you discount water as totally obvious, ask yourself, do you drink enough of it? Chances are the answer is no.

Your body is about 60% water. It needs water for almost every function it carries out from regulating your body temperature, lubricating your joints, transporting oxygen throughout your body, and eliminating waste.

Water is so fundamental that you can survive weeks without food but only days without water.

We now know a healthy gut is essential for healthy skin, but what you might not know is that our gut needs two things to stay in good working order:

1. Fibre
2. Water

Fibre usually steals the limelight when it comes to our

digestive health. Consuming lots of fruit and vegetables will help you to get the required fibre. But without water, fibre can't do its job properly.

Many of us are of the mistaken belief our faeces (sorry, but this is important) are mainly made up of what we eat. This is not true, says Guilia Enders in her book *Gut*. Faeces are three-quarters water and "consuming dietary fibre is little help if you do not also consume sufficient fluids. Without the presence of water, fibre binds together in solid lumps."

Water is a critical component of a healthy gut.

If you look at pictures of celebrities, you'll inevitably see them carrying around massive water bottles at some point. That's because their face is often their fortune, and they know what a difference drinking water makes to their skin.

Prove it to yourself by drinking water consistently for four weeks. You'll soon miss it on the days you don't drink it.

How much water we need to drink in a day is another surprisingly contentious part of healthy eating. Some advocate eight glasses of water a day, but then there are debates about what size the glass should be. There are calculations based on your weight, and adjustments based on your gender, level of activity, and even the climate you live in.

Make it easy for yourself and keep an eye on the colour of your pee. It should be pale yellow. If it's dark, you need to drink more water. You'll quickly figure out how much water you need to be drinking to keep your pee the right colour.

Action:

Get a reusable water bottle. Drink one bottle before lunch and one bottle after lunch. Keep an eye on the colour of your urine. You want it to be pale yellow. If it's dark, drink more water.

4.6 HABIT 6 – PRACTICE MINDFUL EATING

While I'm all about adding in the good stuff, sometimes there will be something in your daily diet that is exacerbating, if not triggering, your skin issues.

You can get food intolerance testing through your doctor. My doctor told me that these tests are indicative. If you get tested, and the test comes back clear, that doesn't necessarily mean you're not reacting to that particular food.

You don't need food intolerance tests, though. Your body already knows which foods it likes and which foods it doesn't. We're just not great at listening to our bodies these days. We prefer to listen to that guy/girl/doctor/nutritionist on Instagram that tells us to eat this and don't eat that.

These social platforms are great for people to share their stories, but the only way to understand how particular foods affect your unique body is to listen to it.

Listen to your body

I believe our bodies communicate with us. For people with acne, eczema, and psoriasis, our body uses our skin to talk to us.

Some people's bodies talk to them through their blood pressure, through migraines, heartburn, or that heart attack they suffer in their forties. Even once your skin is healed, it will continue to talk to you, so listen.

I don't believe you can cure acne, eczema, and psoriasis to the point where it will never come back. If the conditions are right, it might come back. But you can get your healthiest skin by optimising your lifestyle for good health. Managing your lifestyle can also make flare-ups less likely and certainly less severe if they do happen.

If you've not already done the skin story exercise, please do it. This exercise helps you see what was going on in your life when your skin was at its worst. It can give you valuable insight into the lifestyle you had, so it's easier to spot when that lifestyle might be creeping back in.

I have this tiny patch of skin on the inside of my left calf. The skin is no longer inflamed, it looks the same as every other patch of skin on my leg. But if I've been eating too much rubbish or not sleeping well, that spot will start to tingle. The tingle begins in the same place. This is where my eczema started. With an itch and one tiny patch of red skin. That patch got bigger then another patch appeared and another until the lower half of my left leg was covered in round patches of rough, flaky, and weeping skin. I had a few patches on my right leg, but the left was always the worst.

As long as I make sure I'm eating well, sleeping enough, and moisturising my skin, the tingle goes away. On the rare occasions when I don't listen, or if I'm ill and I'm not sleeping or eating particularly well anyway, the skin will get red and my eczema will flare-up.

After one particularly gluttonous Easter, I had a flare-up that covered much of my left leg and a small section of my right. It took months to clear and was totally not worth it for a few too many Easter eggs.

I'm much better at listening to my skin these days. I choose not to ignore the warning signs, and I've not had a flare-up as bad as that one since.

When I feel that tiny patch of skin on my leg getting itchy, I listen to it. I see it as a helpful reminder that I need to keep an eye on my lifestyle. It encourages me to take a minute to reflect on what's going well and what needs to be tweaked.

By adding in lots of the good stuff, you'll naturally reduce your intake of foods that may be causing inflammation in your body. This makes it so much easier to identify when a particular food is causing you issues.

Getting started with mindful eating

A more structured way of identifying where you may have issues is to use a mindful eating diary. You can download a template from www.thelifestylecircle.com/bookbonuses or use a notebook and track your eating for a couple of weeks.

Here's how to get started with mindful eating:

- Eat what you usually eat. There's no point in trying

to remove gluten, dairy or whatever else from your diet at this point. You could be cutting foods out unnecessarily.

- Write down everything that you eat and drink each day.

- Set yourself a reminder for 30 minutes after you eat or drink then stop, think about how you feel and write it down.

These questions may help you:

- Are you energised/tired/exhausted?
- How does your stomach feel?
- Are you bloated?
- Do you have cramps/gas/indigestion?
- Are you hungry again?
- Do you feel comfortably/uncomfortably full?
- Are you thirsty?
- Are you craving something sweet/salty/something else?
- Do you have any aches or pains?
- Has your skin broken out?
- Does your skin itch?

Other factors influence how you feel on a daily basis, such as how much sleep you've had, how much water you've had to drink and how much exercise you've done. Note these things too.

I recommend keeping a diary for at least two weeks. You'll then start to notice patterns.

What jumps out at you?

Do you crave sugary foods on days when you've had less sleep? Is milk giving you stomach cramps? Do raw veggies make you bloated? Is bread bunging you up? Do you eat more when you're stressed? Are you shocked by how little water you're drinking? Are you regularly having seconds? Are you snacking constantly throughout the day? Are you just overeating?

Keep things in perspective

One thing I would say when you're completing this reflection exercise is that it's important to keep things in perspective. We all tend to focus on the foods we wish we hadn't eaten.

Chocolate is a regular feature in my mindful eating diary. If it appeared at every meal, I might be worried, but it doesn't. If there are a few things in your mindful eating diary that you wish weren't there, keep it in perspective. Think the 80/20 principle. What you do most of the time has a more significant impact on your health than what you do some of the time.

Pay particular attention to how you feel after eating dairy, gluten, sugar, eggs, and nuts, which can cause issues for some people. We'll look at gluten and dairy in more detail soon.

Remember that people can be sensitive to the most random of ingredients. If you begin to notice a pattern between a particular food and any unpleasant side effects, it's time to revisit your doctor to see if there's further sensitivity testing that might be helpful.

Action:

Go to www.thelifestylecircle.com/bookbonuses to download the mindful eating diary template and start writing. Review your mindful eating diary every couple of weeks and look for patterns.

If you notice a pattern of unpleasant side effects following particular ingredients, discuss it with your doctor. You may choose to avoid those ingredients for a while until your gut health is in better shape.

4.7 HABIT 7 – FAST FOR 12 HOURS EVERY DAY (13 HOURS IS EVEN BETTER)

Before you panic, this one isn't as bad as it sounds.

I was chatting to a friend of mine one day, and it quickly became apparent we were having two completely different conversations. Not only was he not answering the questions I was asking him, but he was rambling incoherently.

Seeing the confusion on my face, he said, "Sorry, it's my fasting day.".

He was doing the Intermittent Fasting Diet. While the Intermittent Fasting Diet works brilliantly for many people, I know it wouldn't work for me. I need to eat. I wouldn't ramble with this style of eating; I would just straight up pass out. So don't worry, this is not the kind of fast I'm recommending!

The 12-hour fasting period I'm suggesting you try is so much easier. Firstly, you're asleep for 8 hours of it. Secondly, you're not missing any meals.

The idea is you eat within a 12-hour window, something Dr

Satchin Panda, in his book *The Circadian Code*, calls Time-Restricted Eating.

Your circadian rhythm

The circadian rhythm is your body's internal clock. Every organ and cell in your body has its own circadian clock meaning it's programmed to carry out its function at certain times of the day or night. In the same way that the sun rises and the sun sets, your body works optimally when it follows the pattern nature has designed your cells to follow. Dr Panda's work demonstrates that the function of our digestive system is also circadian.

Many studies into time-restricted eating focus on weight loss, hence the multitude of fasting diets out there. Studies have shown that people who eat in a shorter window will lose more weight than those eating the same number of calories over a longer period.

To test their time-restricted eating theory, Dr Panda and his team carried out studies on groups of mice. They replicated the high fat/high sugar diet that they say 11,000 other publications had shown caused serious diseases.

When their mice were fed this high fat/high sugar diet within a time-restricted eating window, they did not develop any of the diseases seen in previous trials. They also did not gain excess weight and had normal blood sugar and cholesterol levels.

One explanation for this is the effect time-restricted eating has on the gut microbiome. The study revealed that friendly microbes flourished under time-restricted eating while microbes associated with obesity and disease were suppressed.

Another fascinating aspect of Dr Panda's work is what should happen in our gut when we're asleep.

Daily repair of our gut

We know that our gut provides a home for the microbes that do so much to keep us healthy. We also know that our gut is where we digest our food. Something we've not yet touched on is the daily maintenance needed to keep our gut in tip-top shape.

Our gut is lined with tightly packed cells that prevent the contents of our gut from getting through to our bloodstream. When any of those cells become loose or damaged they allow particles of undigested food through, triggering a response from our immune system and creating inflammation in the body.

This is called increased intestinal permeability or leaky gut, which I mentioned earlier, and can be caused by gut infections, use of antibiotics, poor diet, misuse of alcohol, and/or food intolerances.

What I found so interesting in Dr Panda's work is that he says damage to our gut is to be expected and occurs every day. It's estimated that 10 to 14% of the cells in our gut need to be replaced each day. This repair process is circadian, meaning when we sleep our body gets to work to repair any damaged cells.

If this is the case, we need to give our gut the time and space to do its nightly work, which it can't do if we're constantly asking it to digest food. If regular late-night eating happens, your gut lining will remain in this compromised state keeping your immune system on high alert as it deals with the contents of your gut leaking out. This creates unnecessary inflammation in your body and triggers, or exacerbates, issues on your skin.

Time-restricted eating

Eating within a smaller window gives your digestive system enough time to digest your food, repair and rejuvenate the gut, and supports the growth of beneficial bugs in the gut, processes that are interrupted or incomplete when your digestive system is dealing with a constant influx of food.

But why a 12-hour fast?

Dr Panda and his team ran their experiments in 8, 9, 10, 12, and 15-hour windows. The benefits associated with time-restricted eating were observed in those eating within an eight to 12-hour window. The health benefits they observed from eating within a 12-hour window doubled at 11 hours and doubled again at 10 hours.

A 12-hour window is achievable for most people so start there. Once you're consistently eating within a 12-hour window, drop it to an 11-hour window and see if you experience any additional benefits.

Action:

Be mindful of when you are eating. Eat all of your meals within a 12-hour window so you're fasting for the other 12 hours.

4.8 HABIT 8 – SNACK LESS

The world is made up of two types of people; those who snack and those who don't. I'm a snacker. If you are too, you're probably thinking that this section of the book will be utter nonsense that you'll never be able to do. But I promise, once you've read this section, you'll never look at a snack in the same way again.

Just in case the fear of not eating snacks is distracting you too much to pay attention to what you're about to read, let me say right up front that you don't need to do this straight away. Always take the path of least resistance. If snacking less feels like it would be the hardest habit for you to crack, don't bother tackling it until you have some of the other habits under your belt.

To snack or not to snack

When I was 21-years-old, I fainted in an elevator. I remember feeling a heat building up inside of me, my stomach churning, my heart racing, and sweat appearing from nowhere. I was just about to leave work anyway, so I grabbed my bag and headed for the elevator. One of my colleagues, also on his way home, joined me, and as soon as the doors closed, I felt myself go. My head hit the metal floor, and everything went dark.

When the elevator reached the ground floor and the doors opened, I can only imagine the sight, my shocked colleague and me unconscious in a heap on the floor. I worked in a hospital, and the person on the other side of the door was a doctor. I was literally driven across the car park in an ambulance, where I sat in Accident and Emergency for a couple of hours before I was allowed to go home.

This wasn't the first time I had fainted, nor was it the last. It also wasn't the last time I knocked myself out by hitting my head. Probably explains a few things!

Fainting was a regular occurrence for me. I fainted in school, in university, and in multiple workplaces.

Despite doctors' visits, trips to A&E, and multiple blood tests, no one was ever able to say why I fainted. The only advice I was given was to keep snacks handy because snacks would keep my blood sugar levels stable.

I followed this advice and became a snacker. My typical eating pattern was breakfast, lunch, dinner, two snacks, and copious cups of tea every day.

I continued to faint until I was in my late twenties. I still have no idea why, and I have no idea why I stopped fainting. Perhaps, by the time I was 30, I had finally outgrown fainting. Not that I'm complaining. My point is, we sometimes do things, like eating snacks, for the right reasons. The rationale makes total sense. But there's another way to look at snacking that makes just as much sense.

Do we need to snack?

No, is the answer. Our ancestors never snacked. Our grandparents never snacked. Depending on how old you are, your parents might not have snacked either. They ate their three meals a day, and that was it. Snacking is a recent change in our eating habits, and snacks have become a billion-dollar industry.

You can find plenty of scientific studies that show snacking is a good thing, and find plenty that show it isn't. Some studies show that snacking keeps our blood sugar levels stable and stops us from binging on food later. In contrast, others show that constant snacking keeps our insulin levels artificially high, which causes us other problems.

There's no definitive view, so I don't think of snacking as good or bad. It's just something most of us do. And hopefully, it goes without saying that snacking on a banana is far better for you than snacking on a couple of chocolate biscuits.

What interests me more about snacking is the effect it has on our digestive system.

How often do you eat?

How often have you eaten today, or yesterday if you're reading this in the morning? Not how much you had to eat, but how often you ate.

For many people, a typical day involves breakfast, then a

coffee/tea, and a snack mid-morning. It's then lunchtime, followed by another coffee/tea and snack mid-afternoon and perhaps the odd biscuit, handful of nuts or sweets throughout the afternoon. Dinner is then often followed by more nibbles while watching TV and maybe a glass of wine or gin and tonic.

Many of us are grazing all day, and eating six or more times a day means your digestive system is not getting a chance to finish digesting breakfast before it has to fire itself up again to deal with the snack you've just sent its way.

On top of this, if you're then snacking close to bedtime, you're disrupting your circadian rhythm and affecting the nightly cell renewal process in your gut, compromising your gut lining.

I'm going to share something with you that will change the way you look at snacks.

Let your housekeeper do her job

While we might not understand why certain bodily functions are important, there's one thing we do know, there's a reason our body does everything even if we don't yet understand the reason.

Most digestion and absorption of nutrients takes place in the small intestine. This is where your food is broken down into particles that are small enough to be absorbed into your bloodstream and lymphatic system.

An extra little bit of homework now. Watch the TED talk by Giulia Enders called *The Surprisingly Charming Science of your Gut*. Giulia says, when your stomach rumbles, it's not because you are hungry. It's because your small intestine is a neat freak and wants to use the time between digesting one meal and the next to clean everything up.

Any undigested or unabsorbed matter needs to be swept into your large intestine. This 'sweeping' is a process called the 'migrating motor complex', nicknamed by scientists as 'the housekeeper'. It's this muscle movement that can create the rumbling sound you hear in your gut.

The housekeeper wants to keep the small intestine spick and span, but she can't start work until the stomach and small intestine are empty. This is perhaps why we associate our tummy rumbling with being hungry.

Next time your tummy rumbles, don't immediately grab a snack. When you eat, the housekeeper has to stop work, regardless of whether or not the clean-up is complete.

Snacking all day leaves little chance for your housekeeper to do her job, meaning your digestive system is not functioning as it should.

One easy way to help your housekeeper out, according to Giulia Enders, is to create less work for her by chewing your food well.

Digestion begins with your eyes. Your stomach produces digestive juices on sight in anticipation of the food it's about to receive.

The next stage of digestion is chewing. Your teeth and digestive enzymes in your saliva break down the food you're eating until you swallow, sending it on its way to be further pulverised in your stomach before it reaches your small intestine.

Chewing is a much-undervalued part of our digestive process. You'll find some gut health experts recommend chewing your food up to 30 times. Whether it's 10 times, 20 times or 30 times, I don't know. But there's a good chance it's more chews than you're currently doing. So get chewing. You're aiming for your food to be pretty mushy when you swallow it.

Taking the time to understand a little more about what's going on inside you changes how you think. And when you think differently, you behave differently.

If you're a snacker like me, chances are you hear your tummy rumbling and you reach for a snack. Now that you know what that rumble actually means, you might instead think, "should I eat this snack? Nah, best not. That's the housekeeper about to start cleaning, so I'll just wait till lunchtime.".

How to snack mindfully

I'm not saying don't snack. I'm saying snack less. Become more mindful of your snacking habits, know what's going to happen inside your body when you eat that snack and decide if you still want it. Sometimes you do, and that's OK. But let's stop the mindless snacking that we've become accustomed to.

Start by chewing well then, next time you feel the urge to snack, ask yourself a few questions:

- Is it worth firing up your digestive system all over again?

- How long do you have to wait until your next meal? If it's not long, can you let your housekeeper finish her clean-up and distract yourself with something else for an hour or so?

- Are you actually hungry? If so, eat a meal.

The best way to snack mindfully is to eat meals, not snacks. I don't want you to feel deprived, so if you want to eat a bar of chocolate or bag of nuts, eat them. But eat it as part of your meal, not as a snack a couple of hours after your meal. The point is not to deprive yourself of what you want to eat, it's to be a bit more mindful over when you choose to eat so your digestive system (specifically your housekeeper) has the space to do her job between your meals.

Action:

Watch the TED talk by Giulia Enders called *The Surprisingly Charming Science of your Gut*. Give your housekeeper a helping hand by chewing your food well and snacking less.

4.9 HABIT 9 – EAT REAL FOOD

One of the best ways of getting a variety of healthy food in your diet is to eat real food. To quote Jamie Oliver, "Real food doesn't have ingredients. Real food is ingredients.".

That means cooking.

Cooking doesn't need to be complicated three-course meals that take an hour of prep and an hour of cooking. It can be as simple as baking a potato, steaming a piece of fish, stir-frying a pile of vegetables, and chopping a salad. But if cooking to you currently involves boiling a pot of pasta and putting something on a baking tray ready for the oven, even these simple cooking suggestions can seem daunting.

Many of us don't cook for one of two key reasons:

1. We believe we can't cook. No one teaches us to cook. It's not something we learn in school. All I remember making in Home Economic classes in school were cakes and cheese on toast. And if you

didn't learn to cook at home, you won't learn unless you take action to teach yourself.

2. We're overwhelmed. There are quite literally millions of recipes online for free. You can find out how to make anything and everything within a few seconds. While you might think this would be a good thing, what often happens is that we end up spending hours on the Internet trying to find something to cook. We waste so much time we don't then have time to cook it, so we end up having pesto pasta again because we're too hungry to wait for anything else. Just me?

Cookbooks are the answer to both of these challenges.

How many cookbooks do you have in your house? If you're like most people, chances are it's more than one. Also, if you're like most people, you've likely not cooked more than a handful of recipes from them.

To learn to cook, I went back to basics and used the cookbooks I have in my house. Following a recipe is cooking, and there are recipe books out there for every level of cooking expertise, from absolute beginners to the more adventurous cooks.

Using the physical book means the number of recipes you're flicking through is limited to what's in the book. You're not getting lost down an Internet rabbit hole. Once you get started, you'll soon find you begin to use the cookbooks for meal inspiration, not necessarily instruction. You'll go from following full recipes to the letter to finding something you fancy, then adding stuff to it or tweaking the recipe when you don't have all of the ingredients.

If the thought of preparing a full meal in the kitchen makes you break out in a sweat, make it less threatening by involving others. Ask a friend to help or get your family involved. You'll have a bit of a laugh, and you'll be teaching your family valuable skills that will stay with them for life.

Make it a bit more fun by doing something else while you cook. When I'm cooking, I usually have an audiobook or podcast playing along in the background. Or, if I'm home alone, I have '90s music blaring out of my iPad. There's nothing like a bit of Alanis Morissette to take the edge off my time in the kitchen.

Remember that cooking doesn't have to mean hours in the kitchen. There are many short cuts available to us, some are helpful, and some are not.

The convenient kitchen

If you look around your supermarket, you'll find a handful of aisles of fresh produce. The rest of the supermarket is ready meals, cereals, cakes, biscuits, crisps, and fizzy drinks.

These are 'foods' made in a factory using lots of ingredients, many of which are not good for us. Even something as simple as a loaf of bread can now contain upwards of 15 plus ingredients. We've lost the basic recipe of flour, water, salt, and yeast.

We've become consumers that value convenience. But as the population becomes increasingly overweight and unhealthy, we're becoming increasingly health-conscious consumers too.

These convenience foods have nutritional information labels on them that tell us how many calories we're about to consume, the recommended portion size, how much salt, sugar, and fat are in the product.

Those same products have marketing messages on the front that claim the product counts as one of your five-a-day, is low in saturated fats, heart-healthy, contains 25% less sugar, a good source of vitamin D, under 100 calories, suitable for vegans, amongst other claims.

Real food doesn't have these labels. It doesn't need them.

It's easy to say that the solution is to stop eating processed food. But it's hard to do this. Most food has an element of processing. We're not plucking the chickens and shelling the peas ourselves, are we?

Developing a better appreciation of how to navigate the world of convenience food, which, let's face it, isn't going anywhere, is more helpful.

Let's look at some simple ways of eating real food that still allows you to benefit from the convenient kitchen.

Prepared versus Processed

Learn to recognise the difference between something prepared for convenience and something processed with additives, emulsifiers, flavourings, colourings, sweeteners, and preservatives.

Have you ever chopped a whole pineapple? It's such a

nuisance, but it tastes amazing. Occasionally I buy a whole pineapple, but more often than not I buy pineapple chunks that someone else has already prepared for me. I buy the pineapple from the fridge or freezer section of my supermarket with the ingredients listed as "pineapple".

I avoid pineapple in the tinned section because it contains "pineapple, pineapple juice concentrate, sugar, ascorbic acid, and natural flavouring". Despite the manufacturer telling me that their pineapple is freshly packed in 100% juice and a rich source of vitamin C, I don't want it. I just want pineapple, without the other stuff.

Pre-prepared fruits and veggies can be a great way of getting variety in your diet. You can now readily buy prepared butternut squash, mango, pineapple, riced cauliflower, chopped onions, sliced mushrooms, vegetable medleys, and ready for roasting sweet potato fries. These foods can be a great addition to your diet when you're confident that you're getting only what it says on the front of the packet.

The only way to tell is to flip the packet over and read the ingredients.

Ingredient consciousness

Ignore all of the marketing messages on the front of packaged food and look at the back of the packet instead. Getting in the habit of reading labels is a simple way of making healthier choices. If you recognise the ingredients as food, eat it if you want to. If you don't recognise the ingredients as food, put it back.

If you were making the product at home, would you use the same ingredients?

I took a look at two different pre-prepared chicken soups. If you were making chicken soup at home, you likely would add chicken, stock, and veggies, which were the main ingredients in one of the soups. But it's unlikely you would add dried milk powder, milk proteins, polyphosphates and sodium phosphates, which were the added ingredients in the second soup.

I love dips. I top salads with them, and I dip vegetables, nachos, and oatcakes in them. I go for shop-bought hummus because my supermarket stocks one made from chickpeas, tahini, oil, lemon juice, salt, and garlic. All ingredients I recognise and things I would use at home if I made it.

I make my own guacamole by mixing mashed avocado, lime juice, crushed garlic, and chopped tomatoes. The supermarket guacamole contains potato flakes, whey extract, whey powder, sugar, dried glucose syrup, glucono-delta-lactone, dextrose, chlorophyllin to name only some of the added ingredients. Except for sugar, I have none of the other ingredients in my kitchen.

Convenience is great when you're clear what you're getting and what you're getting is real food.

My message here is to minimise foods with a long list of ingredients and minimise foods that have ingredients you wouldn't use at home.

Free-From doesn't mean good for you

Free-From foods can be a lifeline for people with food allergies and intolerances, we'll talk more about that later on, but the quality varies hugely. Pretty much anything printed on the front of a packet food is marketing. There's no point wasting time reading it.

Take a look at many of the cereal boxes these days and you'll see a large percentage of them are proudly shouting that they're vegan-friendly. A high sugar, high salt, high fake-food cereal doesn't contain much goodness, whether it's vegan-friendly or not.

Your supermarket probably has a 'wellbeing' or 'free-from' aisle. It'll be full of products claiming to be gluten-free, dairy-free, sugar-free, or free-from something else. But if you stop and look for a minute at this aisle, you'll see it's a collection of cereal, bread, pasta, cakes, biscuits, crisps, and drinks. Highly processed foods with a long list of ingredients that you wouldn't use at home.

We'll come back to this topic, but for now, don't assume something in the wellbeing aisle means it's actually good for your wellbeing.

Action:

Gradually build up your confidence in the kitchen. Cooking will help you to get in the habit of eating real food. Get one of your cookbooks and commit to making one of the recipes every other weekend. When you're taking a short cut, choose prepared over processed, and read ingredients.

4.10 WHAT TO DO NEXT

There you have them, the nine habits that finally brought me relief from acne, eczema, and psoriasis.

To recap, the habits are:

1. **Fall in love with food** again by making some new good food memories.

2. **Banish the Beige** and brighten up your meals.

3. **Eat 20 – 30 different varieties** of fruits and vegetables each week. Print off your free tracker from your book bonuses and increase the varieties you eat gradually.

4. **Use the 80/20 principle** in your diet and lifestyle.

5. **Keep an eye on the colour of your pee.** It should be pale yellow. If it's dark, drink more water.

6. Practice mindful eating. Download your free mindful eating diary template from your book bonuses.

7. Fast for 12 hours every day (13 hours is even better) to give your gut a chance to carry out its nightly repairs.

8. Snack less and chew your food more to give the housekeeper in your gut a helping hand.

9. Eat real food. Minimise foods with a long list of ingredients and minimise foods that have ingredients you wouldn't use at home.

You might be saying 'is that it? All I have to do is throw some extra veg on my plate?'. In short, yes. The point of this book is to help you to give the bugs in your gut what they need to thrive so they, in turn, can help you to thrive. They're really not that demanding. If you feed them a variety of fruits and vegetables and drink water to keep your digestive system ticking over, they're happy.

The habits are straightforward but that's why they work so well.

Feeling a bit overwhelmed?

If introducing these habits seems like too big a leap for you given where you are now, don't worry, I'm going to help you get started in a way that's doable regardless of where you are now.

I started off eating four or five varieties of fruit and vegetables a week, in a good week, so I've learned a few hints and tips for making the change and avoiding overwhelm along the way.

Part six of this book looks at how you can make a sustainable change to your eating habits, so these habits become just the way you eat.

Starting can be the most difficult bit of any habit change. I won't lie and tell you this is going to be easy. But it will be much easier than you think.

PART V

FREQUENTLY ASKED
QUESTIONS

5.1 WHAT'S THE DEAL WITH SUGAR?

It seems impossible to talk about health these days without demonizing sugar. You might be surprised to learn that I don't stress about sugar too much.

I cook most of my meals, don't drink many fizzy drinks, eat lots of fruits and vegetables, and drink plenty of water. Therefore I don't worry too much when I eat a bag of chocolate buttons, sweet popcorn at the cinema, or an almond milk chai latte from Starbucks.

If you're relying on convenience food, you're snacking on sugary biscuits, and you're drinking six cups of tea a day with two spoons of sugar in each one then, yes, we do need to talk about sugar.

I'm talking about added sugars here, not the natural sugars found in whole foods such as fruit. I don't buy into the narrative that sugar found in fruit is bad for us. Nature has helpfully packaged the sugars found in fruit with vitamins and other beneficial nutrients. Fruit is also a good source of fibre, essential for a healthy gut.

A diet that's high in added sugar and low in fruits and vegetables causes the microbes in your gut to starve. If you're eating many so-called simple carbohydrates or starchy foods, things like bread, pasta, white rice, and other snacks and meals that are high in sugar and low in fibre, then this is an issue for you. These foods behave like sugar in that they are absorbed into the bloodstream in the small intestine. Most of your microbiome is in your large intestine.

This means that what you're eating is not reaching your large intestine, so it can't provide food for your microbes. Your bugs are literally starving.

But, bacteria are right up there as one of the most adaptable species, hence why they've lived for billions of years.

In their book *Gut Reactions*, scientists Justin and Erica Sonnenburg say that when your gut bacteria don't have what they need to eat, they adapt. Rather than go hungry, they will instead feast on the mucus layer that lines your gut. This creates the conditions for leaky gut, which can trigger a reaction from your immune system and cause inflammation in the body and on the skin.

The short story on sugar is that we all need to consume less of it. Reducing your intake of packaged and processed foods will greatly help here.

When you're eating bread or pasta, think about what you can add to your plate that will feed your microbiome. Fruits, vegetables, or a simple salad is all you need.

Another easy way to reduce your sugar intake is to ditch the fizzy drinks.

While I usually focus on adding in lots of good stuff to your diet to heal your skin, this is one of the few things I recommend cutting way back.

There's nothing in a fizzy soda that your body needs. It's just sugar and artificial sweeteners. There's nothing of any substance in a fizzy drink.

If you can't ditch the fizz altogether, decide that you'll only drink them when you are out for dinner. Turn your daily habit into a weekly or monthly habit. Choose a non-alcoholic cocktail in place of your usual soda to make that fizzy drink something special rather than something you rely on to quench your thirst.

Sugar is not good for us. We all know that. If you can cut it out completely, brilliant. If not, like me, do what you can to reduce your intake. Preparing your meals with real food will help you to do this.

5.2 IS ORGANIC HEALTHIER?

A question I often get asked is whether or not it's healthier to eat organic produce.

There's no consensus on whether or not eating organic has any health benefits. There are certainly environmental and animal welfare benefits to organic farming, so it's worth exploring for those reasons alone.

With fruit and vegetables, I don't worry too much about getting organic produce. There's not a great variety of organic fruit and vegetables in my local supermarkets.

If you prefer the idea of organic fruit and vegetables, keep an eye out for the Environmental Working Group's annual list of the dirty dozen and clean fifteen. It's a list of the fruits and vegetables found to have the most and the least pesticide residue.

I prefer to eat blueberries even if they're not organic. I wash them thoroughly and tuck in.

That said, I will gorge on whatever fresh produce is in

season and will always choose local versus imported if there's a choice between the two. A trip to a local farm for Pick Your Own fruit and vegetables is a great family day out, and the produce tastes amazing when it's fresh, seasonal, and local. I love seeing kids wandering around with muddy wellies and strawberry-stained smiles.

Where I will prioritise organic is meat, eggs, and dairy. I'm lucky living in Scotland because much of our cattle and sheep are outdoor-reared and grass-fed. I always opt for local rather than imported animal produce.

According to the Soil Association, organic farming has the highest animal welfare standards of any international farming system. With organic farming, the animals have a better quality of life, their diet is better, and they have had less exposure to antibiotics and growth hormones. There are debates about whether these antibiotics and hormones end up in the produce, which in turn, end up in you. For me, it's just not worth the risk when there are alternatives.

It's worth taking the time to look at farming practices wherever you live. Choose local, grass-fed, organic animal produce wherever possible. Yes, it will cost you more. But you're likely to eat less of it, which will help you create more space in your diet to eat more vegetables.

You don't need to be vegetarian or vegan to have glowing skin. But the quality of the meat you consume is important.

5.3 DO I HAVE A FOOD INTOLERANCE?

When I speak to people about their skin, the big focus is usually on what they can remove. That's a tiny part of the puzzle in my experience. Eliminating foods from my diet had little effect. It wasn't until I started adding in lots of healthy foods that my skin began to heal.

Don't worry about removing things from your diet unless you know you're reacting to a particular food. This book's focus is to get you eating enough of the good stuff to make sure those microbes in your gut are well fed.

Should I just cut out gluten and dairy?

It's hard to go anywhere online these days without someone advocating for a gluten and dairy-free diet. And many people living with acne, eczema, or psoriasis choose to minimise gluten and dairy, particularly those that also have gut symptoms.

Too much dairy is a problem for me, but I saw little

improvement in my skin when I first tried removing dairy from my diet.

As my diet became more diverse, I naturally ate less dairy. It wasn't long before I noticed that my stomach would feel uncomfortable, and my skin would itch on the days I ate dairy.

I decided to try an elimination diet. I just excluded dairy and gluten since these were the two things I suspected may have been causing me an issue. I couldn't shake the feeling dairy was a problem for me despite my lactose intolerance test being negative.

I'd tried elimination diets unsuccessfully in the past, but there was a crucial difference this time. I wasn't substituting dairy with soya, and gluten with processed foods. My diet was much more varied.

I substituted dairy milk with almond milk, and I laid off cheese, yogurts, and chocolate. My diet was no longer reliant on toast and pasta, so cutting gluten out for a short period was no hard-ship. My skin continued to improve, and my IBS settled.

These days, I minimise dairy in my diet because I feel ill if I have too much. I eat gluten, but I choose good quality over quantity.

I told a doctor about my experience with dairy. He said that this sounded very typical of lactose intolerance. He also said that the hospital tests are only indicative, and the best way to tell for sure is to remove the suspected food from your diet for a short time and monitor how you get on. I was a bit annoyed to hear this after being repeatedly told food wasn't an issue, but, hey, I got over it.

Cutting out gluten and dairy is unlikely to heal your skin if you're not also adding in the good stuff that your gut needs to be healthy.

The best way to enjoy gluten and dairy

I don't believe there's anything inherently bad about gluten and dairy. But I do think we're all eating far too much of it. Reduce the quantity and increase the quality, and you might find gluten and dairy don't cause you any issues.

Increase the quality

Make sure you're eating the best quality gluten and dairy. For example, eat fresh bread from the bakers rather than the processed sliced white. You want the type of bread that goes hard if you don't eat it within a couple of days rather than the kind that goes mouldy if you don't eat it after a week.

Your issue with bread might not be gluten or wheat. It might be the other crap they put in the bread to give it a longer shelf life.

If you still find it's causing you an issue, don't assume gluten-free bread will be better for you. Take a look at the list of ingredients and you'll often find it's long with ingredients you don't recognise as food.

If you're eating yogurt, eat natural or Greek yogurt and sweeten it yourself with fruit and a little honey or maple syrup.

Experiment with different types of cheese and, it sounds obvious, but make sure it's cheese. There are lots of products in the fridge masquerading as cheese but are not. They are products with a small percentage of cheese bulked out with water, oils, preservatives, and flavourings.

When you reduce the quantity of gluten and dairy in your diet, you create space for a wider variety of all the good stuff.

Instead of having buttered toast every morning, you might have it once or twice a week. On the other days, you might have an omelette with tomatoes, mushrooms, greens, and a sprinkling of chopped chives, a green smoothie stuffed with spinach, banana, and berries, a bowl of fresh fruit salad with yogurt and granola, or porridge oats topped with fruit, nuts, and seeds.

Not all gluten and dairy are equal

You might find you can tolerate parmesan cheese on your pasta or Greek yogurt with your fruit, but drinking a glass of milk or a latte is a no-no.

A couple of slices of sourdough bread might be OK, but rye bread causes you heartburn.

Experiment and see what works for you. Find your limits.

It's also useful to regularly check in with yourself. If you react to gluten and dairy, it might be because your gut is not in great shape. Once your gut is healthier, you may find you're better able to tolerate gluten and dairy.

If not, and you're still reacting to gluten and dairy, don't worry about cutting them out. Gluten is not essential to anyone's diet.

Reducing or eliminating dairy tends to be the most contro- versial, not for the individual who sees and feels a dramatic difference, but for their friends and family. It's not the first time someone has told me that reducing my dairy intake is bad because I'll not be getting enough calcium.

There are many non-dairy ways to ensure you're getting enough calcium such as fish where you eat the soft bones (e.g. tinned salmon, tinned sardines, whitebait), leafy greens, tahini, chickpeas, almonds, brazil nuts, dried apricots, and broccoli.

If you're worried about missing out on gluten and dairy, I encourage you to read *The 4 Pillar Plan* by Dr Rangan Chaterjee. Dr Chaterjee says, "Misguided commentators in the media have portrayed the avoidance of gluten, and dairy, as some sort of dietary fad, as if they are somehow essential food groups. They are not. There are several populations around the world who consume little to no dairy, such as the Chinese, and do just fine.".

About food substitutions

Remember my philosophy of 'what you eat matters more than what you don't eat'.

If you find you're intolerant to dairy, you're not going to see much of a difference if you substitute chocolate biscuits for free-from chocolate biscuits. There's nothing in a chocolate biscuit, even if it is gluten and dairy-free, which will nourish your gut.

If you're going to try dairy-free, try different types of dairy-free milk. When I first made the switch, I went for soya milk, but my skin and gut issues remained. I now know soya has the same effect on my body as dairy, which is common.

Almond, oat, hemp, and rice milk are readily available in many supermarkets.

Look for brands that use only ingredients you recognise so you're not getting a load of nasty fillers too.

Remember habit 9 – eat real food. If you can't readily buy the ingredients in your supermarket, put it back on the shelf.

How to tell if you have a food intolerance

The first step is to speak with your doctor. You can be referred for tests to check your reactions to common food groups. Just remember that these tests are indicative.

Practising mindful eating (habit 6) will help you narrow down your symptoms and possible food-related triggers. If you're looking to take this further, you can do an elimination diet.

An elimination diet involves removing possible trigger foods from your diet for four weeks, then adding them back in, one at a time, and monitoring for any reactions.

Just remember that removing foods alone is unlikely to heal your skin.

Focus on enriching your diet first, eating lots of fresh, healthy foods, and drinking lots of water before considering food restrictions.

Once you're eating a healthy, colourful and varied diet, if you still believe food may be a trigger for your skin, I recommend then trying an elimination diet. It's the best way to tell how your particular body reacts to certain foods.

Elimination diets are safe because you are removing foods for a short time only.

Just make sure you get the all-clear from your doctor before starting an elimination diet.

Common triggers to remove during an elimination diet are:

- Dairy
- Gluten
- Sugar
- Eggs
- Soy
- Fast food
- Alcohol

If a particular food is negatively impacting your health, you should feel better having removed it from your diet for those 4 weeks.

One by one, add in the excluded foods and note any reactions. Reactions may take a couple of days to appear, so it's important to reintroduce the excluded foods individually.

If there's no reaction, you can reintroduce the food into your diet and move on to another excluded food until you've successfully reintroduced all of the foods.

If you notice symptoms after reintroducing a particular food, talk to your doctor again. They can help you make sure you're not missing any key nutritional elements while avoiding the food that's causing you issues.

A reaction to a food doesn't mean that food needs to be excluded for life. You may be better able to tolerate previously excluded foods when the health of your gut is better.

An elimination diet can be tough, especially if your diet before starting it is beige.

Focus on getting a healthy gut first by feeding your microbes what they need to thrive. Once you're consistent with this, you'll see clearly the foods that make you feel good and the foods that don't and may not even need an elimination diet to tell you this.

5.4 WHAT CAN I DO WHEN I GET A FLARE-UP?

Firstly, look out for warning signs and actually listen to them. Next, ask yourself what's new or different in your life.

Most of us are creatures of habit. We typically do the same things, go to the same places, eat the same foods, and meet the same people on a weekly, if not daily, basis. This can be helpful for people struggling with a skin condition. The routine makes it easier to identify the new thing that might be a trigger for your skin issues.

I've heard people say the following:

- I've been so busy at work I haven't been eating very well.
- I always break out when I get my period.
- I've not slept much this week thinking about my big presentation on Friday.
- I've been snacking on lots of nuts this week.
- I used a new moisturiser / cleanser / facemask.
- I was away for the weekend and had lots of wine.

Spending a few minutes thinking about what's new or different in your life can pinpoint what might be triggers for you. Once you've identified the possible trigger, it's easier to put a plan in place to minimise the chance of that trigger continuing to cause you problems.

Where there's a clear trigger, such as a new product you've been using, it's easier to deal with. You stop using that product.

When it's something a bit more complex, such as, 'I've been so busy at work I haven't been eating very well', this is where you need to spend time working out a plan to deal with the situation in a way that minimises the impact on your skin.

I've outlined some actions in the next section of this book to help you be busy and still eat well. There will always be aspects of your lifestyle that you won't feel in control of at all times. Modern culture seems to celebrate busy. If you're not busy, you're not working hard enough, you're lazy or have an easy life. I don't think this is healthy, and we should try to find ways to make our lives less busy. But that's a subject for another book.

Even if we find ways to slow down, there will always be busy periods, so it's important to plan for those.

As I said earlier, I don't believe you can cure acne, eczema, or psoriasis to the point where it will never come back. Your body communicates with you through your skin, so flare-ups are almost inevitable. When they happen, reflect on the warning signs.

With the benefit of hindsight, were there signs you didn't at first realise were there? What was going on in your life that may have contributed to your flare-up? What steps can you take to minimise that being a continuing factor?

The more you learn about your unique body, how it works, and what other factors influence it, the happier you will be in your own skin and the fewer flare-ups you'll have.

PART VI

CHANGING YOUR HABITS

6.1 CHANGING YOUR HABITS

If you think reading the nine habits and understanding the theory behind the habits is enough to get you motivated to eat well for life, think again.

How many things have you said you want to do if you could just get yourself motivated?

Eat healthier food if you could just get motivated to cook. Get fit if you could just get motivated to go to the gym. Get a new job if you could just get motivated to update your CV. Write a book if you could just get motivated to start writing.

Motivation has a habit of disappearing right when you need it most.

What you need is to make a decision, then make a plan. Once you've made a decision that you want to do something, start planning it. Don't rely on motivation or willpower, or you just won't do it. Writer Mel Robbins says, 'you will never ever feel like it'.

Think of it like a holiday. You decide you want to go to New

York on holiday then you start planning it. You research when and where; you book the flights and you go.

Decide you will introduce one or more of the habits in this book, make a plan about how you're going to do it, and start doing it. Let the rest of this book help you create the plan so you can start today.

Decide now that you want to change your eating habits then use the system in this book to make it easy for yourself to do it until the changes become the way you do things.

Motivation might get you started on day one, but motivation is not enough to keep you going. We are all creatures of habit. The only way to make a lasting change is to change our habits.

6.2 CHANGING OUR HABITS IS CHILD'S PLAY

Have you ever noticed that habits are easy to form but hard to change?

While considering how to change our eating habits, I wondered why, if habits are easy to form, they're so difficult to change.

We continue to form habits throughout our lives, starting when we're tiny babies. We cry when we're hungry, and someone comes along and gives us food. We learn to cry to get what we want. When we're a bit older, we learn to point to what we want, then learn to ask for what we want, then we start helping ourselves.

Many of our eating habits form in childhood. Sure, our tastes change a bit as we get older but how healthy our diets are, whether we cook, if we have breakfast, and where and when we eat are usually habits that stem back to childhood.

In looking at how our habits form in childhood, I wondered if we can use the same tools and techniques we use with children to change our habits when we're all grown up.

What our kids teach us about changing our habits

When our children are young, we do some key things to help their development and influence their behaviour. If you're a parent, you'll recognise all of this.

- **We celebrate the baby steps.** When my daughter took her first step, I was over the moon. I was cheering her on to try more and giving her lots of praise for the one tiny step she took. With our children, we recognise the importance of that one step. It's one step closer to their goal of being able to walk. We don't expect them to walk the full length of the living room, let alone run a mile. When we're first encouraging them to walk, we don't stand at the opposite end of the room and expect them to come to us. We stand an arm's length away. Taking things one step at a time will get us where we want to go.

- **We encourage them to try, try, and try again.** When our children are learning to walk or ride their bikes, we know it'll take time. They'll fall over sometimes, and that's OK. Whereas we tell ourselves, it's useless, and we'll never change when we miss one yoga class or eat a bar of chocolate. Can you imagine doing that with your child when they're learning to walk? They take a step and fall over. You'd never respond with "it's no use, you'll never be able to walk, you may as well stop trying now.". Failing is a natural part of doing something new, and that's OK.

- **Everything gets tracked.** When our children are tiny, their height, weight, speech development, and walking are tracked as key milestones. Even their bowel movements get tracked when they first come home from the hospital. The reason for this is to keep a close eye on progress. As long as they are hitting established mini-goals or steps, they're thriving. We all accept there's a curve along which they'll develop, but as long as they're making progress, we know they'll eventually get where they need to be. Trackers work, and they encourage us to take it one step at a time.

- **Rewards work, but it has to be the right reward.** We don't reward our children for their good behaviour by allowing them to run wild for an hour. We know this would undermine everything we've been encouraging them to do. Yet with our diets, how often have you rewarded yourself for sticking to your healthy eating habits with a takeaway or a piece of chocolate cake as a reward for the bowl of salad you've just eaten. This type of reward doesn't work because it undermines the new habits you're trying to foster. Kids respond well to stickers on a chart, buttons in a jar, or ticks on a list. When we do give them a treat, it's something different from the behaviour being rewarded. For example, we don't reward them for sleeping in their own bed all night by allowing them to sleep in our beds at the weekend. But we might reward them by buying them a magazine or a trip to the cinema. This type of reward acknowledges the work they're doing and encourages them to continue with it but, crucially, does not undermine the behaviour we're trying to promote.

- **Everyone has an off day.** When I was weaning my daughter, I was advised to monitor her food intake over a week rather than a single meal or day. This made sense and stuck with me. She was hungrier on some days than others and was more inclined to try new foods on some days than others. As long as she was eating a healthy balanced diet across the week, I didn't stress about individual meals or snacks. Promoting a healthy balance is a better approach than setting unrealistic expectations. Think habit 4 – the 80/20 principle.

- **We're mindful of the way we talk to them.** We give them tough love when they need it, but most of the time, we're supportive, compassionate, and kind. We're encouraging, and we praise them for the things that have gone right rather than dwelling on the things that have gone wrong. We can apply this same principle to our eating habits by congratulating ourselves for what's gone well instead of focusing on the one or two things that didn't go quite as hoped.

- **We teach them moderation.** We don't allow our children to binge-eat. We do our best to make sure they're getting a balanced diet. We wouldn't let them eat a whole box of cookies in one sitting or only have chips and dip for dinner. We teach them they need to eat proper meals before they get

snacks, and snacking is in moderation. Habit 8 –
snack less.

- **We don't give our kids the weekend off from good
  behaviour.** We expect good behaviour all of the
  time. It's easy to fall into the trap of being "good"
  during the week then, by implication, allowing
  ourselves to be "bad" at the weekends. I've done
  this myself, but it can be a harmful way of thinking
  about eating. Changing our language around this
  might look like a subtle difference, but it can be so
  powerful. Habit 4 – the 80/20 principle encourages
  us to think differently about our eating choices. We
  all know there's little nutrition in cookies, cakes,
  and commercial chocolate bars. But it's unrealistic
  to tell yourself you'll never eat these things again.
  You're not 'being bad' by eating cake. As long as
  you're eating a wide variety of healthy foods, eating
  a piece of cake now and then can also be a healthy
  choice. Giving yourself a day off is what you do
  when you're on a diet. You're not on a diet. You're
  someone that eats a wide variety of healthy food —
  every day.

- **We don't wing it.** With our kids, we don't usually
  wing it. We spend time learning a set of tools that
  we can use depending on the situation. We watch
  Supernanny and read some of the tens of
  thousands of parenting books out there. We learn
  techniques for time out, the naughty step, sleep
  techniques, and the best ways to potty train. That's
  why this book encourages you to take specific

actions and make a plan, so it's easier for you to make healthier choices every day.

- **They add before they subtract.** When we teach our kids maths, we start with 1 + 1 = 2. We teach them to add before we teach them to subtract. Adding is easier. Once they get the hang of adding, we then teach them subtraction. It's the same with our diet. It's far easier to add things to our diet than it is to take them away. People get put off making changes because they hear the word change, and they automatically think it means stop. It's hard to stop things we've been doing for a long time, if not all of our lives. The habits in this book, such as habit 2 – Banish the Beige, focus on adding lots of healthy habits to the way you eat, not taking foods away.

I've taken these parenting principles and built them into the habits and action steps outlined in this book. I've created a supporting habit change framework that's easy to understand and works to get you results.

Let's look at the strategies you can use to make the nine eating habits in this book easy for you to adopt in your life.

6.3 EMBRACE YOUR COMFORT ZONES

People tend to talk about comfort zones like they are a bad thing. We're taught that pushing ourselves outside of our comfort zone is good, that we learn best and achieve more when we get outside of our comfort zone.

But what if there is also another way to look at comfort zones? What if we can use our comfort zones to our benefit?

When we operate within our comfort zone, we do so without much thought. Our everyday behaviour is automatic. We don't stress about it, and we don't make decisions, we just do it. Much of our time in a day is spent operating in our comfort zone. It's what we do and, for the most part, what we've done for a long time. It makes us feel safe and contented.

We can use our comfort zones to our advantage when changing our habits.

If you've tried to change your eating habits in the past, you've likely gone on a diet. You may have eaten better for a few days or a few weeks, but, at some point, you've come off the diet and reverted to your previous way of eating. Whatever changes you made were not sustainable because you were following someone else's diet plan.

You may have been faced with ingredients you've never heard of, recipes you're not familiar with, food you don't like, and a heap of other rules to follow. You didn't make any changes to your habits.

The eating habits in this book don't ask you to change your routine or get rid of things from your diet. They ask you to add things, one step at a time. By adding things, you gradually stretch your comfort zone. You make your comfort zone ever so slightly wider at a pace that doesn't freak you out. You're allowing yourself to win at the habit change game every day.

Let's look at skydiving as an example. It's a pretty random example, but definitely an activity that's most people would describe as out of their comfort zone.

For many of us, skydiving is so far outside our comfort zone we'll never do it. But you hear of people that do it once, find it so exhilarating they immediately book up for another dive. They experience an immediate rush and are desperate to experience it again. There's no learning curve. There's a short safety talk then, on the same day, they get strapped on to an experienced instructor and away they go, plummeting through the sky at 120 miles per hour. Skydiving doesn't just take you out of your comfort zone; it obliterates your comfort zone in minutes.

Changing your eating habits is on the opposite end of the spectrum from this.

You don't see any benefits from eating a portion of broccoli.

You don't get a rush of good feelings, your digestive system doesn't immediately thank you, and your skin doesn't suddenly glow. You will get these benefits, but only if you consistently eat broccoli and other vegetables over a longer period.

For this reason, it can be better to edge your way out of your comfort zone rather than trying to obliterate it in one day.

Making dramatic changes to your eating habits isn't exhilarating for most of us. Most of us will feel the natural pull to get us back into our comfort zone, and we'll struggle to maintain our new eating habits.

Comfort zones are neither good nor bad. We all have comfort zones, and we all react differently when our comfort zones are challenged.

I'm going to ask you to look at the first steps you will take to make the eating habits in this book your new eating habits.

In determining your first steps, your job is to find that sweet spot where you feel challenged but not overwhelmed.

6.4 START SMALL

A journey of a thousand miles begins with a single step.

Lao Tzu

Your first step depends on your starting point and your tolerance to change. Some people change quickly. They decide one day they're going to do something, and they do it. They make big changes all at once, and those changes stick.

Given you're reading this book, I'm assuming you're like me, and habits are a bit more challenging to make and break. In that case, starting small is what you need.

You might decide to start with one habit, or choose two or three habits to start. You might even decide to try a single step within each of the nine habits simultaneously. There's no right or wrong. There's only the way that works for you.

Remember that you're looking for that sweet spot where you feel challenged but not overwhelmed. When you're about to start something new, it's easy to get overwhelmed. Your initial enthusiasm wanes after a few days or a few weeks, and you give up. Usually, this happens because you're trying to do too much too soon.

Being healthy is a process, not a single event. Long-term change is what we're after. It's far better to take it slowly and make lasting changes than try to get there too fast and struggle to maintain it. Be the tortoise rather than the hare.

The smaller the step, the more likely you are to do it. And when you do it, you feel good about it and keep going.

S J Scott, in his book *Bad Habits No More*, says, "the best long-term results come from making gradual changes in your life.". You form the habit first then gradually expand that habit until you're where you want to be.

Keep your first step so tiny that it's completely doable for you. Practise that step consistently, then add in another small step, and another one, and you'll soon see progress.

That tiny step might be eating one extra fruit or vegetable in a day. It might be eating a handful of spinach with dinner every night. It might be drinking one extra glass of water. If so, this is fine. It's better to start where you are rather than where you think you should be to make lasting change.

Don't underestimate the power of starting small. Remember that we're borrowing from the techniques we use to teach our children. Children learn their lifelong skills by repeating small steps. They learn to walk one step at a time, talk one word at a time, eat well one food at a time, and sleep in their own beds one night at a time.

As parents, our job is to set their environment up to allow them to achieve these little wins consistently. With consistent action, momentum builds, and they take more steps, say more words, eat more food, and sleep longer. They quickly build on those initial steps and get where they need to be.

That's exactly what you'll do too. You'll decide on those first steps you'll take, then you'll make incremental upgrades to those steps over time.

Your job right now is to design your environment to allow yourself to achieve little wins consistently. What will your first step be, and when will you complete it? Choose the best time in the day to start.

Breakfast is often a good one because it's when your willpower muscle is at its strongest. But if mornings are a manic rush for you with screaming kids, packed lunches to make, and homework to find, you will struggle to have the best breakfast. Dinner might be a better option if you're calmer and less harassed.

Inevitably some of the habits will be easier for you to stick to than others. If you find yourself struggling to stick with a habit, wind it back a bit. You might be trying to do too much too soon.

Action:

Decide right now what your small step is going to be. Now decide when you'll do it. Remember to add before you subtract. Make your small step adding in good foods rather than changing what you perceive to be bad.

I found it helpful to focus on upgrading my diet, not depriving myself of what I enjoy.

We'll come on to accountability later, which you might need to make sure you actually do it.

6.5 FOCUS ON THE SYSTEM, NOT THE OUTCOME

Your desired outcome might be to get glowing skin, feel healthier, heal your gut, or get rid of your constant heartburn. These are all great health goals, and can be achieved by changing your eating habits. But for a minute, let's forget about these desired outcomes.

In researching making and breaking habits, I came across the work of James Clear. James talks about focusing on the system, not the goal.

If your goal is clear skin, it's easy to get disheartened every day that your skin is not clear. But if you're focusing on the system, and that system is eating well, you get to celebrate each time you eat a healthy meal. You celebrate the baby steps. Your choices every day become a reason to celebrate - how great is that?

Forget about your bigger why for a moment. Keep your focus on the baby steps. If you focus on "I'm eating well to heal my skin," when your skin isn't healing after two days, one week, one month, you give up and say it's not working.

To get the benefits of healthy eating, you have to eat that way for life. You're not going to eat well for a month, heal all of your ailments then return to current eating habits. That will achieve nothing. Remember it took time for your skin to get to its current state and it will take time for it to improve.

Your goal is to eat well for life. Stop focusing on the longer-term goal and focus on the step that's right in front of you.

Being healthy is not something you achieve and tick off the list. It's something you have to do every day. Changing your habits and being healthy becomes something you no longer have to work at, it becomes something you do and the way you are, and that's when you'll see the greatest results.

View the plan you commit to as the system. Focus on that system, not the outcome. Small steps that build over time will always get you life-changing results.

6.6 JUST START, AND DON'T STOP

5-4-3-2-1-go. This is the five-second rule from Mel Robbins. Mel says the moment you have an instinct to act on a goal you must physically move or your brain will stop you. We all know that cooking a healthy meal from scratch is better for us than pressing start on the microwave. But sometimes just the thought of pulling out the chopping board is too much for us and it's easier not to do it.

The simplicity of Mel's five-second rule is that you never give yourself a chance to talk yourself out of it. Mel says that the five-second rule activates your prefrontal cortex, which is the part of the brain responsible for decision making, learning new behaviour and working towards goals. When you count then physically move, grab the pan, or grab the chopping board, you've started. Continuing is much easier than starting.

When I was trying to get in the habit of exercising, keeping my first step small was key. I committed to exercising for two minutes every day. Everyone has two minutes. It was such a small goal that I had to do it. More often than not, those two minutes would turn into a lot longer, and my exercise habit had begun.

There's not a week goes by now that I don't do some form of exercise. Although admittedly, it's still easier some days than it is others. For those days when I just don't feel like it, 5-4-3-2-1-go is what gets me going.

Once you've decided on your first steps, just do them. And if you're struggling, think 5-4-3-2-1-go and move.

Just as important as getting started is not stopping.

When we're teaching our children something, whether that's to walk, talk or tie their shoes, we don't let them stop. Even when we see them struggling or they fall over, we encourage them to try and try again. It's the same with our habits. There will be days when it feels easy, days when it feels hard and days when we want to throw in the towel altogether.

In the book *Willpower* by Roy F. Baumeister and John Tierney, the authors cite studies showing something researchers call Counterregulatory Eating, or the What-the-Hell Effect. The research showed that when dieters considered that they'd blown their diet for the day, they considered the whole day to be a failure and, saying what-the-hell, overate for the rest of that day. The same principles apply to those trying to eat a healthier diet.

A friend of mine was trying to lose weight with the 5:2 fasting diet. For 5 days of the week she was eating normally and, on the other 2 days, she was fasting by restricting her food intake to 500 calories.

Her husband came home on one of her fast day evenings

and found her tucking into a takeaway and an Easter egg. 'I ruined my fast day by having soup at lunchtime, so I figured I may as well eat today and fast tomorrow instead'.

She used one bowl of soup to rationalise her decision to have a takeaway and an Easter egg on a Tuesday night. This is the what-the-hell effect in action. The only next step she had in her mind was to try again the following day.

This is why the 80/20 principle and healthy follows unhealthy works. When you're eating well, you're taking it one meal at a time. You don't stop eating well regardless of what your last meal was. Everything you eat is an opportunity to reset your day.

Not stopping can be especially helpful for holidays. If you've been on a diet before, then you know how the story goes. You eat well for weeks or months, then a family holiday, or often Christmas, ruins it all.

You stuff yourself with endless turkey dinners, bacon rolls, and chocolate. You succumb to the what-the-hell effect, and you end up eating this way all week. The only vegetable that passes your lips is that Brussels sprout you feel obliged to eat.

The beauty of my approach is that you absolutely have permission to pig out on turkey and stuffing. That's the 20% in your 80/20 principle. Ditch the language of starting and stopping diets or being on and off plans. When you stop or come off something, it's harder to get back on track. But you follow the 80/20 principle, so you never need to stop. It doesn't matter if one particular week that principle is more like 65/35. You never need to stop eating well; you just might need to tweak your ratio now and again.

6.7 MAKE THE HEALTHIEST CHOICE THE EASIEST CHOICE

It's vital to make any new habit easy. Most of us are a delightful combination of pretty lazy and pretty busy. If trying something new seems like hard work or is too time-consuming, then we'll likely never start it let alone practice it consistently until it becomes just how we do things.

Unless you love cooking, you'll probably want to make your meals in the time it takes to boil some pasta and stir through a spoon of pesto. Here are some ideas to keep mealtimes quick:

- **Embrace the wok** – stir frys can take 10 minutes.

- **Sunday meal prep** – take some time on Sundays to set yourself up for success the rest of the week. You can go all out, cook all of your meals and store them in the fridge and freezer ready for the week ahead. Or keep it simple and just roast a chicken (or buy one ready roasted), roast a big pan of vegetables, slice some raw vegetables, cook rice and boil eggs.

Store everything in the fridge and you have the basic ingredients to pull together a quick meal as soon as you get home from work.

- **Have a standby meal in mind** – for me, this is pasta. There are always those days where you can't be bothered. I keep a bag of brown rice pasta and a jar of pesto in the cupboard. Probably once or twice a fortnight, I will make a batch of pasta for dinner. I make it healthier by loading it with vegetables and serving it with a handful of salad greens. This is also a great one to do at the end of the week to use up any leftover vegetables to minimise food waste.

- **Use your freezer** – when making meals, make extra portions to stick in the freezer. When you know you'll be having a late night or a busy day, just take your meal out of the freezer and warm it up. The other thing I use my freezer for is storing frozen fruit and veg. I always keep peas, sweet corn, green beans, berries, pineapple, and bananas in there. This way, I have ingredients to hand to make a smoothie for breakfast or to add vegetables to my meals at night when I can't be bothered chopping or have nothing fresh in the fridge.

- **Cook once, eat twice** – when you're cooking, get in the habit of cooking extra portions. It takes very little extra time and you'll have tomorrow's dinner already made meaning you're not cooking every night.

- **Plan your meals** – when you know what you're

going home to cook for dinner, you're more likely to do it. It's often standing dithering in front of the fridge, unsure what to cook, that leads to unhealthy choices.

- **Eat the same meals on set days a week** – while I'm all about variety, it helps me to know what I'm cooking a few nights of the week. For example, I always make salmon on Wednesdays. I serve the salmon with whatever vegetables or salad I bought that week. Sometimes I have it baked with lemon juice, other times I'll have it with tamari, ginger, garlic and honey, other days I'll have it with pesto and sometimes I'll cook it with tamari and apricot jam (so good, don't knock it till you've tried it).

- **Keep salad dressings simple** – most of the time, I serve my salads with black pepper and extra virgin olive oil, lemon juice, hummus, pesto, or feta cheese. These dressings are minimum fuss and full of flavour.

Action:

Write down how you can make eating well easier. Use the examples above for inspiration.

6.8 MAKE THE HEALTHIEST CHOICE THE VISIBLE CHOICE

Part of making healthy eating easier is making the healthy choice the visible choice. We've already talked about how busy people are these days. Unless we've planned in advance, we tend to open the fridge and make our dinner choices based on the limited amount of food we see.

An easy switch is to get in the habit of keeping the healthiest food visible and the unhealthy stuff hidden away.

- In your fridge, keep the healthiest food visible. Fruit and vegetables are usually hidden away in salad drawers at the bottom of the fridge. When you open the fridge, you want to see an abundance of colours to whet your appetite for more of the good stuff.

- Store leftovers in glass containers. As with your fruit and vegetables, you want to see in an instant what healthy food you already have available to you. If you're tired and hungry, you'll open the fridge and see healthy leftovers you can eat in minutes. If your leftovers are not obvious, you're more likely to open the fridge, see only foods that take a bit of effort to prepare and reach for the plain pesto pasta instead.

- Change the position of your fruit bowl. If you stock your fruit bowl then throw away mouldy peaches and brown bananas at the end of the week, it might be that your fruit bowl is just blending into your kitchen décor. Change where you keep your fruit bowl. You'll notice it again and will be more likely to eat its contents.

- Put biscuits, cakes, and sweets out of sight. Don't buy the unhealthy foods, put them at the back of the cupboard, on a high shelf, or inside a storage container where you can't see them. Make unhealthy foods less visible and put healthier foods at eye level with maximum visibility.

Action:

Write down how you can make healthy food visible in your home and work environment.

6.9 SUMMARY OF THE HABIT CHANGE FRAMEWORK

- **Aim to gradually stretch your comfort zone** when it comes to eating well. You want to feel challenged, not overwhelmed.

- **Add before you subtract.** Focus on adding in the good rather than trying to change what you perceive to be bad. You're upgrading your diet, not depriving yourself of what you enjoy.

- **Keep your changes small** so you do them consistently. Keep adding more small steps until you get to where you want to be.

- **Focus on the system, not the outcome.** Every time you complete your small step you're winning, and making progress towards your bigger goals.

- **Just start, and don't stop.** Don't consciously give yourself time off from your new habits. You'll find it hard to re-start. You will miss a step at some point.

Just pick it back up again at the next opportunity, and you're still on track.

- **Make your new habits easy to do.** Write down ways you can make eating well easy for you. Use the examples in this book to help you.

- **Design your environment** to make fruit and vegetables more visible.

Action:

Go through each of the habits. Decide where you'll start. You might want to commit to one or two habits or choose a small step within every habit. Remember that there's no right or wrong, and everyone has a different starting point.

Decide on your first small step. Keep it small so it's achievable for you every day. You'll then look at incremental upgrades to keep you making progress within each habit. If you find you're struggling to consistently practice your habit, make your first step even smaller until you're getting consistency again. Remember, you should feel challenged, but not overwhelmed.

Decide when you'll complete your step. You want to set yourself up to succeed, so don't choose a time you know will be a struggle.

Write down how you'll track your progress. You can find my monthly calendar template in your book bonuses. Print it out and just tick every day that you complete your first, or next, steps. There are several electronic habit trackers you can download if you prefer digital.

Some of these habits will be easier for you to do than others. If you're finding one particularly challenging, focus on some of the easier ones first. If needed, get some extra accountability by asking a friend or family member to help monitor your progress, or invest in coaching.

Go to www.thelifestylecircle.com/bookbonuses to download and complete the My New Habits table, or grab a notepad and create your own table with the following headings:

- Habits 1 – 9
- Start now or later
- Small first step
- When
- Tracking method
- Extra accountability, if needed

Complete the table then get started. And don't forget to have fun! Think of yourself as a bit of a science experiment. Do the work, and you'll learn a lot about what works and what doesn't for you, which you can carry forward to every part of your life.

PART VII

OVERCOMING OBSTACLES

7.1 OVERCOMING OBSTACLES

I hope what you've read so far has inspired you to start making some changes to your eating habits. But to stop this from being the type of book you follow for a few days then give up with because it's too hard, let's consider all of the things that might derail your attempts to build your new healthy eating habits.

It's not a lack of knowledge that prevents us from improving our diet. Despite the billion-dollar diet industry, most of us intrinsically know eating more vegetables and drinking more water would improve our health. What stops us from doing this is one or more perceived obstacles that we struggle to see a path around.

This is why the final part of this book is overcoming obstacles.

An obstacle is simply a thing that is making it more difficult for you to do something, in this case, eat a healthier diet. But obstacles can almost always be overcome.

Consistency is so important when building new habits. But

sometimes it feels as though life is conspiring against you. Sometimes it kind of is, and sometimes it's just an excuse you're making for yourself.

Thinking in advance of what might knock you off track and how you'll overcome that is extremely helpful in keeping you going.

To quote Marie Forleo here, "Everything is Figureoutable". If you stop and think about it, there's a way around pretty much everything that might try to stop you from following your new habits.

We're going to look at how to overcome the obstacles that might show up for you. Before we do that, I've listed below the most common obstacles I have heard people say. I've also listed some solutions to each obstacle.

Obstacle 1 – Getting started

Sometimes the biggest obstacle is just getting started. Anything new takes you out of your comfort zone. We've discussed that the tools in this book keep you inside of your comfort zone. Sometimes people still need to be told the first step then they're off and running. If you're someone that needs a step-by-step guide, this book is it. I've included a handy action list at the end of this book and a printable version in the book bonuses. All you need to do is follow the action list, step-by-step. Read the action list, and you know exactly what your first step is.

Obstacle 2 – Other people's opinion

The topic of food can be contentious these days. Everyone has an opinion on other people's food choices.

What I've learned through 10 years of doctors, nutritionists, and naturopaths is the only person that can tell me how my body reacts to a particular way of eating is me.

You might hear some of your friends and family saying things like:

"Go on, life's too short, have a dessert."
"You're so boring."
"Ugh, you're not going veggie, are you?"
"Eating veg is your latest fad then is it?"
"All that green stuff is for cows, not people."

Seriously, people can be that rude.

Here are a few specific solutions that work well when dealing with other people's opinions.

- Other people's opinions of you are none of your business. Lots of variations of this quote exist online, and I can't find where it originated, but it fits well when it comes to healthy eating.

- It's not you, it's them. Other people's opinions are usually driven by *their* feelings over *their* choices. They might be trying to make themselves feel less self-conscious about their choices by getting you to indulge with them. Or perhaps they're reacting to you making positive changes in your life because it reminds them that they're not. Whatever the reason, their opinions usually say more about them than they do about you.

- Have a few stock phrases on standby that you can reel off whenever someone challenges your food choices. For example, "I've been eating a healthier diet over the last few weeks and I feel so much better that I'm sticking with it", "I've been making the effort to eat more veg and I feel great so I'm going to keep it up", "I feel better than I have in years but thanks for your concern" and a simple "No, thank you, I'm so stuffed I wouldn't enjoy it".

- You're not on a strict diet, so if you truly want dessert, have it. But make sure you're eating it because you want too rather than because you're succumbing to peer pressure. Remember your 80/20 principle.

Once you feel amazing because of your new healthy eating habits, other people's opinions stop bothering you so much. In fact, other people will comment on how well you're looking, and you'll delight in telling them what you're doing and why.

Obstacle 3 – I'm too busy

OK, be honest with yourself here. How much time do you spend watching TV in the evening? Whatever it is, it's OK because we all need a bit of downtime. But can you commit to only watching a particular show in the kitchen, so you're watching it and prepping a healthy meal at the same time?

Or record your favourite show so you can fast forward through the adverts and use the extra time to make a healthy meal.

Is 'I'm too busy' secretly code for 'cooking is boring'? If so, ask your partner to sit in the kitchen with you while you prepare meals (or even better, help you to make the meal) so you can spend some time together while you cook.

Make cooking something you look forward to by listening to music, a podcast, or audiobook as you cook.

I understand the busy obstacle. Everyone is too busy these days. But you owe it to yourself to start taking better care of yourself. You're reading this book because you're not happy with your health, whether that's your skin, your gut or something else. You can change that, but you're going to have to make some changes to do that.

Go back and think about your first small step. Make the first step a tiny step that doesn't take you more than a few seconds so you can do it regardless of how busy you are. Here are some examples of tiny steps that take seconds:

- Wash an apple and eat it.
- Peel a banana and eat it.
- Add some frozen peas and sweetcorn to your pasta or rice as it cooks.
- Line your bowl with a handful of leafy greens from the fridge and put your usual dinner on top.
- Add a handful of fresh herbs to the top of your meal.
- Wash a baby cucumber and eat it.
- Crush a couple of garlic cloves into your meal as it cooks.

- Wash some sugar snap peas, dip them in hummus and eat them raw.
- Sprinkle a tub of edamame beans onto your meal.
- Buy a salad rather than a sandwich when you're out for lunch.
- Order the dish on the restaurant menu you think is likely to be the most colourful.
- Order a side salad with your meal in the restaurant.

There's always a way to do something, no matter how busy you are versus not doing it all.

How to deal with busy periods

Regardless of how well we're doing with our new eating habits, there's always an even busier than usual spell that comes up for us that we know will make it difficult for us. The best way to deal with this is to spend some time in advance of the busy period planning how you can be busy and still eat well.

To give you some ideas, you can:

- Spend some time the weekend before filling your freezer with healthy meals you can defrost and warm up when you get home.

- Roast a chicken and a tray of vegetables on Sunday so you can eat it for lunches all week.

- Give your partner your chosen menu for the week and ask them to prepare the meals.

- Share cooking with a friend. She cooks one dish, and you cook another. She gives you a portion of her meal, and you give her one of yours. This is a tip I picked up when I was weaning my daughter. It meant less cooking but a greater variety of meal options in the freezer.

- Investigate healthier meal delivery services in your area. Sometimes outsourcing the work for a short period is the best option.

- Find a couple of meals you like that you can make in minutes. Mine is miso soup. I simply slice up raw veggies (sugar snap peas, spinach, carrot, peppers, spring onions), add hot water from the kettle and a tablespoon of miso paste for a quick and tasty soup. Sometimes I add pre-cooked rice, or vermicelli noodles, which just soften in the water.

- Use the standby meal we discussed in 'make the healthiest choice the easiest choice'. My standby meal is pasta. I can have dinner ready to go in 10 minutes by boiling pasta, adding a load of vegetables from the freezer and mixing through a spoon of pesto.

- Fill your desk drawer with healthy snacks, so you always have something to hand when hunger or stress gets you. Nuts, seeds, oatcakes, and dried fruit are good options.

- Cook once, eat twice. When you're cooking, get in the habit of cooking extra portions. It takes very little extra time, and you'll have tomorrow's dinner already made meaning you're not cooking every night.

- Plan to fail but plan how you'll get back on track too, so you know exactly what to do next.

- Follow the 80/20 principle. Sometimes it's OK to be busy and have takeaway food. Give yourself a break.

Obstacle 4 – I don't have any fruit and vegetables in the house

We've all been there. Our intentions are good, and we go to the fridge to see what we can add to our meal, and it's bare. The best way to avoid this is to use the freezer. Frozen fruit and vegetables mean you'll always have some to hand, even when you haven't been to the supermarket.

Obstacle 5 – I'll need to go to the supermarket every other day and eat weird stuff

I remember watching some of those diet programmes from the noughties where people were trying to slim down or get rid of their cheeseburger addictions. They were usually given diet plans with ingredients like buckwheat, quinoa, sauerkraut, mung beans, and alfalfa sprouts. Ingredients you're not sure how to say, let alone where to find, in the supermarket.

Part of the show was watching them trying the foods like they were kids being asked to eat jellied eels.

By the way, I love some of these foods now, although I'm still not sure what a mung bean is! Anyway, the biggest gripes on these shows were they didn't recognise the foods, and they had to go to the supermarket more often to buy the fresh foods they were being made to eat.

You can get around the supermarket issue two ways:

- Buy softer fruits and vegetables for the beginning of the week and hardier varieties to keep for the end of the week. This is also a great tip to minimise food waste.

- Keep a good supply of fruit and vegetables in the freezer so you've always got something you can add to your meals without having to shop every other day.

Obstacle 6 – Money

There's a perception that eating well is more expensive. It's unfortunately true that it is cheaper to buy a portion of fries or a sandwich than it is to buy a pot of fresh fruit. That said, there's a supermarket to suit every price range. In fact, many of the so-called cheaper supermarkets are seeing a huge upturn in customer numbers as people of all budgets get fed up with the ever-increasing price of food.

With meat and eggs, I buy local and organic wherever I can. For everything else, it just depends on the availability. I choose local over imported where I can, but I live in Scotland, foods like pineapples are not grown here.

Frozen vegetables are often cheaper than fresh and are just as nutritious.

I don't stress about buying organic because it's often not available. Eating non-organic vegetables is better for you than eating no vegetables at all.

Obstacle 7 – I love family meals, and I'll feel bad eating different food from everyone else

Remember that you're adding goodness to the meals you already eat. You can still eat the same meals as the rest of your family but with extra goodness heaped on top.

Adding more fruit and vegetables to your family meals is also something that will support the health of your family, so get them in on the act. Make it a family challenge. Support each other or get competitive with it, whatever works for your family.

I find printing a fruit and vegetable tracker for everyone in the family is a great way of getting them to support your new eating habits inadvertently. A little bit of competition over who can eat the widest variety of fruit and vegetables in a week is a good thing. My daughter will eat a vegetable she claims to hate just to put it on her chart to keep her a few veggies ahead of her dad.

As I mentioned earlier, educate your kids about their gut health. Keep it simple and encourage them to see their microbes as little pets living inside of them, and it's their responsibility to feed them every day.

You can also start by choosing fruit and vegetables you think your children will enjoy if they try them.

If all else fails, go back to what you might have done when your kids were weaning, i.e. hide the vegetables in the food.

Add garlic, onions, mushrooms, peppers, tomatoes, carrots, and celery to a pasta sauce, but blend the sauce so the kids don't even know it's there.

If you continue to get resistance, don't let it derail your changes. Serve the fruit and vegetables as side dishes. Your family can then choose to add them, or not, to their meal. I find my daughter is more willing to try new foods when they are served tapas-style in the middle of the table. She can have a good look at it first, and she can take just a tiny bit then choose more if she likes it, which she inevitably does.

Remember that healthy eating habits that feed your gut are as good for your family as they are for you.

Obstacle 8 – I love my food too much to change

This one comes from a place of lack and restriction. You've probably followed diet programs before and felt hungry and pretty miserable. The beauty of these habits is that they get you eating lots of the good stuff. Eating well is not a diet. There's no need for you to go hungry.

Obstacle 9 – No one knows what's healthy any more

There will always be food trends. There will always be different studies simultaneously proving and disproving the benefits of particular foods or styles of eating. What is common to any healthy diet is that vegetables and water are good for you, so just start there.

Once you get a handle on your health by feeding your gut what it needs to be healthy, it becomes much easier to navigate the world of food fads and trends because, quite honestly, you stop caring. You know how great you feel, and that's the only thing you're interested in maintaining.

Obstacle 10 - But it's a birthday party/dinner with friends/Christmas dinner

Just follow the 80/20 principle. Remember that the point of getting in the habit of eating well is to add lots of good things to your diet. It's not saying don't eat cake. If you're at a party and you want to eat cake, eat the cake.

If you're partying at a friend's house, enjoy yourself. Better still, take a salad side dish as a gift to your host.

If it's Christmas, there are so many tasty veggie dishes you can serve with your Christmas dinner. It's not an either-or situation. You can have turkey and stuffing and also have sprouts, parsnips, and cauliflower cheese.

The first habit of eating well we talked about was love your food.

Follow the 80/20 principle by eating healthier before and afterwards, and you can indulge all you like while still giving your body what it needs to keep you in the best health.

Obstacle 11 – I don't like vegetables

My first thought is really, you're an adult, get over it, but I appreciate that's probably not helpful. My second thought is to encourage you to experiment. You will find vegetables that you don't like or don't tolerate well, but you'll find others you love. And you'll love the effect they have on your health and skin.

- Experiment with different types. In my local supermarket, there are six aisles of fruit and vegetables. There must be some varieties amongst them that you like. Buy different types of vegetables each week until you've found the ones you like.

- Experiment with different cooking methods. Roasting is a great method of cooking for those new to veg. You just chop them up and put them in the oven. It's so easy. Roasting also brings out the natural sweetness of the veggies, making them extra tasty.

- Use familiar dips, toppings and sauces. My daughter will eat pretty much anything if there's a spoon of pesto on the side. Enjoy cauliflower cheese, chopped vegetables dipped in hummus, or a teaspoon of pesto mixed in with your cooked vegetables or as a salad dressing.

- Pair those less loved vegetables with familiar dishes. Some people get put off vegetables because they think they'll have to start eating baked aubergine and couscous stuffed peppers. But the best way of broadening the variety of veggies you eat is to pair them with foods that are familiar to you. This is where the LOADED habit comes in. A curry, for example, is an easy dish to make with half meat and half vegetables. You can have pesto pasta that's loaded with extra veg. Or chilli with the usual meat, onions and kidney beans, plus black beans, garlic, red peppers, mushrooms, and grated courgette.

Obstacle 12 – I don't want to waste food

Some people worry they'll buy lots of fruit and vegetables at the start of the week and throw it all away at the end of the week. This was a problem for me before I started to change my habits. I would start the week full of good intentions and fill my fridge with lots of fresh produce. By the end of the week, I'd have a fridge drawer full of squelchy veg fit only for the bin.

As I hope you've learned by now, good intentions are not enough for you to make lasting changes to your eating habits.

Food waste is a real issue but let's find ways to minimise food waste rather than allow it to become an obstacle to you eating well.

I'm certainly not perfect, but here are some of my favourite ways to minimise food waste.

- The best way to minimise food waste is to eat the food. Ground-breaking, I know. Aim to eat all of the fruit and vegetables you buy. Your wallet, the environment, and your health will all thank you.

- Don't overbuy. Buy what you think you'll be able to eat. You can always pop to the shop later in the week if you run out. As your new eating habits become more familiar, you'll soon figure out when you're under or overbuying.

- Eat the softer fruits and vegetables at the beginning of the week and leave the hardier varieties for later in the week. For example, eat your blueberries before your apples and your asparagus before your leeks.

- If you do notice your fruit is getting a bit squidgy, make a smoothie. Or how about making a chia seed jam. Just heat your squidgy fruit in a pan until it's even more squidgy then add a couple of spoons of chia seeds. The chia seeds will thicken it to give it a jam-like consistency. Or bake it in the oven either on its own or as part of a fruit crumble.

- Use your freezer. I always keep a few bags of veg in my freezer so if I run out, and can't get to the shops, I still have the option of vegetables with dinner. You can also freeze any fresh fruit or veg you know you're not going to use before it spoils. Peel and halve bananas then freeze them. Blend them into smoothies or blitz them on their own once frozen to make healthy ice cream. Slice and freeze any leftover fruit so you can add to your next smoothie. Chop peppers, onions and whatever other vegetables you have. Freeze them then add handfuls straight from the freezer to your next stir-fry.

- Buy loose produce. If you're cooking for one or two people, it can be easier to buy fresh produce loose rather than by the bagful. This way, you get a good variety of vegetables without having 15 extra carrots lurking in the fridge.

- My personal favourite is to have a weekly leftovers

dish. One day of each week, I make a loaded veggie pasta, stir-fry, or veggie curry. I add all of the veg sitting in my fridge that I didn't quite get round to eating that week. It's a great way of minimising food waste, and eating a wide variety of vegetables. Plus one day in the week at least you know you're having a healthy meal without much thought or planning.

- Make loaded tomato sauce. Sauté some onions, garlic and whatever vegetables are left in the fridge. Add a jar of passata and bring to a simmer. When the vegetables are tender, blend it until you have a smooth sauce. You can then freeze this in portion sizes and use it to make quick pasta, pizzas toppings, and a base for chilli or lasagne. This is also a great one to do if you're hiding veg from your kids.

Obstacle 13 – I want to change my eating habits, but I forget to use the tools

A crucial part of using the tools is, initially at least, reminding yourself to use them.

If you've tried to improve your diet unsuccessfully in the past, you've likely been relying on willpower or the temporary motivation that comes from following someone else's plan. You've been unsuccessful in the past, which is why you're reading this book. You weren't unsuccessful because you lack the motivation, you were unsuccessful because you lacked the tools that delivered lasting change in a way that's right for you.

There's a way to apply these habits regardless of how much

time you have, whether you love or loathe cooking, you eat in, or you eat out. The habits are the same. You don't need any preparation, you can just start using them.

But you might need to remind yourself to use them in the beginning. We're going to look at ways of reminding yourself of your new habits when we look at accountability.

7.2 ACTION: OVERCOMING OBSTACLES

Your task now is to spend time writing down as many obstacles as you can think of that will stop you from eating well. Then write down what steps you can take to overcome those obstacles. Think specifically about:

- What's the first step you've decided to take to get started with your new eating habits?

- What might stop you?

- What can you do to overcome that obstacle?

- If there's a genuine reason why you can't do something, ask yourself what you can do instead? There will be something else you can do that will still help you to stick to your new habits.

When you stop and think through these obstacles logically, you'll see there's always a way around them. Remember Marie Forleo's words, "Everything is Figureoutable".

Go to www.thelifestylecircle.com/bookbonuses to download and complete the Overcoming Obstacles table, or grab a notepad and create your own table with the following headings:

- An easy first step
- I can't do that because
- I can do that if
- I can't do that but I can do [...] instead

PART VIII

ACCOUNTABILITY

8.1 HOW TO STICK TO YOUR NEW HABITS

First up is reminding yourself of your new habits. Without this, you'll fall back on your current eating habits. Once you've decided on your first steps, when you'll carry them out, and how you'll track them, I encourage you to think about a bit of extra accountability.

Remember that you'll find some of the habits easier to introduce than others. For some, all it might take is a reminder on your phone, for other habits, the tracker on your fridge might be enough.

Only you will know how much accountability you'll need to stick to your plans. And don't be afraid to adjust your levels of accountability as you go.

Here are a few ideas to get you started.

- **Set a reminder on your phone for lunchtime to refill your water bottle** – if you're drinking enough water, you should be ready to refill your bottle by lunchtime.

- **Set a reminder on your phone before breakfast, lunch and dinner to Banish the Beige** – most of us eat at the same time every day, so this is a relatively easy way to remind yourself of your new habits.

- **Carry out a weekly review** – sit down for five minutes at the end of the week and review your trackers. Did you hit your goals? If so, give yourself a big pat on the back that you're one step closer to the changes being habits you'll do automatically. If you didn't, what can you do differently next week?

- **Get some external accountability** – tell a friend or your partner what you're doing and ask them to check in with you each week. It's amazing how a little bit of external accountability helps you to stick to your new habits.

- **Use a calendar to mark your progress** – get a monthly view calendar. Put a tick on the days where you stick to your new habits and leave blank the days where you don't. The goal is simply to get more ticks than blank spaces on the calendar by the end of the month. A calendar is a great visual representation of your progress, and it allows you to see in seconds how well you're doing. I love this one because there's no room for kinda doing something. You either did it or didn't do it. You get a tick, or you leave a blank space. Use a cross if that's easier for you. Psychologically a blank space is better for me than a big X.

- **Choose the right rewards** – make sure any reward

you choose to give yourself is not food-related. Seeing the progress you are making as you mark it off on your calendar might be enough of a reward to keep you going. If you need a more tangible incentive than this, give yourself a day off or a day out, buy yourself a magazine or a new book or take a family trip to the cinema to celebrate the progress you're making as a family.

- **Give yourself a consequence for not sticking with your new habits** – if you don't use the tools for a day or two then that's fine, sometimes life just gets in the way. If you don't use the tools for three or four days then you risk not using them again and never seeing the transformation that can occur when you get out of your diet rut. Until the tools become automatic habits for you, give yourself a consequence if you don't use them for more than two days in a row.

8.2 PLAN TO FAIL…BECAUSE YOU WILL

Before I leave you to get on with your plans and embrace the changes, there's one final thing that's helpful to remember. The only thing guaranteed when you change your habits is that you will fail at some point. This is not a bad thing, and it happens to everyone to varying degrees when they try something new.

Accept that failure is inevitable. The best way to deal with failure is to plan for it. Planning for failure is just making sure you have the tools to get straight back up and try again.

Failure is temporary. Failure only becomes permanent if you stop trying. If you keep getting back up and trying again, then you haven't failed. You've simply had a temporary setback.

When you fail:

- Remind yourself you're following the 80/20 principle. You're not aiming for perfection.

- View yourself as an experiment. You'll find some things that work for you. You'll find other things that don't. That's OK. It's all part of the experiment and all valuable data for this and future habit changes.

- Focus on all the healthy choices you've made over the day/week/month. Go back and look at your tracker and see how much progress you've already made.

- Get right back into action and complete your small step at the next available opportunity.

- Consider if your small step is still too big. The point of setting your first steps small is that you do them consistently. If you're consistently failing, wind it back a bit. Make your small step even smaller so you start winning again.

PART IX

NEXT STEPS

9.1 BEYOND THE BEIGE

While my diet was the thing that had the most significant impact on my skin, it's not the only aspect of your lifestyle that has an effect on your skin.

Taking care of my skin on the outside with a good skincare routine, managing my stress, and moving my body were all factors in getting the skin I never imagined would be possible for me.

I don't write this to make you downhearted about how far this book will take you. I write it to encourage you to recognise that you'll get the best results for your health by looking at your health holistically.

In the same way you can't run away from a bad diet, you can't abuse your skin on the outside and expect that it'll glow anyway because you're feeding it well on the inside.

Additional resources

At the start of this book, I mentioned three additional resources to help you get your best skin quicker.

1. Your lifestyle circle exercise. When we give ourselves the space to listen to our bodies, we know what changes we need to make to improve our health. This resource will guide you through key areas of your life to identify any other aspects of your lifestyle that need attention.

2. A guide to skin types. Eating well had a dramatic effect on my acne. Figuring out my true skin type was the final piece of the puzzle. Spoiler alert – acne-prone skin is not a skin type. This guide will show you why your skincare products might be doing more harm than good and what to do instead.

3. A guide to using an emollient. Emollients are still one of the main treatments prescribed for eczema and psoriasis. In this guide, I share the technique for applying an emollient that my doctor taught me. After years of using emollients with little effect, this is the technique that made a difference.

View these resources as complementary to the changes you'll be making to your eating habits. Don't allow them to become a reason for procrastination or for not taking action on everything else in this book.

Go to www.thelifestylecircle.com/bookbonuses to find these additional resources.

9.2 ACTION STEPS TO START NOW

Those are the tools I used to change my diet, which in turn brought me relief from the acne, eczema, and psoriasis that plagued me for 10 years.

Now it's time for you to take action. Get excited to see what an amazing transformation you can achieve. To help you start, I've outlined my suggested next steps below.

- Give yourself a visual. For the next few days, notice the colour of your plates and the colour of your pee. Notice how beige your current meals are and how dark your urine is. Simply becoming more aware of these two things are useful visuals to help you to want to make the change.

- Shift your mindset from cutting foods out of your diet to adding goodness in.

- Enjoy your food, savour every mouthful and go out of your way to make new food memories.

- Complete the My New Habits table from the book or download from your book bonuses. Remember to work one small step at a time. Don't get overwhelmed. If adding in one extra vegetable is a big enough step for you then, great, do that. The key is to choose a step that feels doable to you to enable you to get started. Stop focusing on healing your skin and start celebrating each healthy choice you make. Give yourself a pat on the back (or a tick on your chart) for each glass of water or portion of vegetables you eat. It really is that simple.

- Decide how you'll track your progress. If it's a calendar, print it off. If it's a habit-tracking app, download the app and set it up. If it's a friend or family member checking in with you, have the conversation with them. What you use to track your habits doesn't matter as long as you track them.

- Decide how you'll get some accountability. Are the tools and trackers enough for you? Do you need some external accountability? If so, ask a friend or family member to check in with you, or invest in coaching.

- Complete the Overcoming Obstacles exercise from the book or download from the book bonuses.

- Print off or create your version of the fruit and vegetables tracker. Put it somewhere that you'll see it regularly. Add each different type of fruit and vegetable you eat to the tracker. Enjoy watching the variety of fruit and veg you eat go from single digits to double digits over the coming weeks.

- Choose a meal to start with from breakfast, lunch or dinner. I usually recommend people start with dinner. For the next week, you will Banish the Beige and add lots of colour to your dinner. Vary the vegetables you use. Make your meal LOADED if that resonates more with you. An easy way to do this is to buy a bag of salad greens. Whatever you're having for dinner, add a handful of greens. You can then add additional colours from there. Start slowly to give your digestive system time to get used to the extra fibre.

- Fill a reusable water bottle. Aim to finish the bottle by lunchtime then refill for the afternoon. Keep an eye on the colour of your pee. It should be pale yellow. If it's dark, drink more.

- Give yourself permission now to use the 80/20 principle in your diet and lifestyle and stop aiming for perfection.

Go to www.thelifestylecircle.com/bookbonuses to download and print these steps as a checklist.

CONCLUSION

Dramatically improving your health can be as simple as keeping an eye on the colours on your plate and the colour of your pee.

Now these thoughts have entered your mind from reading this book, you'll find it hard not to notice the colour of your plate and the colour of your pee. When you're faced with these two visuals multiple times every single day, it becomes easier to take action to change.

If there's one thing I want you to take away from this book, it's what you eat matters more than what you don't eat. Stop focusing on cutting things out and going on diets you know you won't last. Focus instead on adding lots of goodness to your diet. You'll feel better, your tastes will change, and your skin will glow from the inside out.

The tools in this book only work if you use them. Don't let this book be another information product you read then forget about. Take action, and you will see and feel a transformation in your health.

Eating vegetables and drinking water are not revolutionary ideas. This book was not to persuade you that eating well is a good idea. You knew that. This book was to give you new insights (or a reminder) of the effect that eating well can have on your skin, as well as a system to change your existing eating habits so eating well becomes what you do rather than something you aspire to do.

Take action and enjoy seeing just how life-changing a strong foundation of eating well really is.

Go to www.thelifestylecircle.com/bookbonuses to download your action steps checklist and get started today.

Knowing something isn't enough. It's doing something with that knowledge that will change your life.

I wish you well on your skin-healing journey.

BOOK BONUSES DOWNLOADS

Don't forget to download your free printables.

- Action steps as a checklist
- Your first steps printable
- Overcoming obstacles printable
- 30 fruit and vegetables tracker
- Meal planner template
- Mindful eating diary template
- Month to view calendar
- Your lifestyle circle printable
- A guide to skin types
- A guide to using an emollient

Download from www.thelifestylecircle.com/bookbonuses

THANK YOU!

Before you go, I'd like to say thank you for purchasing my book. There are lots of great books in the world, and I'm grateful you chose to read mine.

This is the book I wish I could have read when my skin was at its worst. I hope the habits and my habit change framework help you as much as they've helped me.

If you like what you've read and found it useful, could you please take a minute to leave a review? It would help to increase the visibility of this book, so it can help even more people get their best skin.

I'd also love to know how you're getting on.

Come and say hello at www.thelifestylecircle.com.

Thank you once again.

Claire

REFERENCES AND ADDITIONAL RESOURCES

Roy F. Baumeister and John Tierney, Willpower – Why Self-Control is the Secret to Success, 2011

Dr Rangan Chatterjee, The 4 Pillar Plan – How to Relax Eat Move Sleep Your Way to a Longer, Healthier Life, 2018

James Clear, Atomic Habits – An Easy and Proven Way to Build Good Habits and Break Bad Ones, 2018

Guilia Enders, Gut – The Inside Story of our Body's Most Under-rated Organ, 2014

Environmental Working Group. Clean Fifteen and Dirty Dozen, https://www.ewg.org/foodnews/ (accessed February 17, 2020)

Marie Forleo, Everything is Figureoutable, 2019, Audiobook Edition

Jeanette Hyde Nutrition, "Foods for a healthy gut and why eating rich colours matters", http://www.jeannettehyde.com/blog/foods-for-a-healthy-gut-and-why-eating-rich-colours-matters (accessed December 13, 2019)

Jeanette Hyde, The Gut Makeover – 4 Weeks to Nourish your Gut, Revolutionise your Health and Lose Weight, 2015

Mark Hyman, www.drhyman.com (accessed June 18, 2020)

Cecilia Jernberg, Sonja Löfmark, Charlotta Edlund, Janet K. Jansson, "Long-term impacts of antibiotic exposure on the human intestinal microbiota", November 01, 2010, Microbiology Society, https://www.microbiologyresearch.org/content/journal/micro/10.1099/mic.0.040618-0 (accessed February 03, 2020)

The Lancet. "Over 95% of the world's population has health problems, with over a third having more than five ailments." ScienceDaily, www.sciencedaily.com/releases/2015/06/150608081753.htm (accessed November 27, 2019)

Dr Michael Mosley, The Clever Guts Diet – How to Revolutionise your Body from the Inside Out, 2017

NFU Scotland. Farming Facts. What we produce, https://www.nfus.org.uk/farming-facts/what-we-produce.aspx (accessed February 17, 2020)

NHS Oxfordshire, "Calcium for bones – in a dairy free diet", https://www.ouh.nhs.uk/osteoporosis/documents/calcium-for-dairyfree.pdf (accessed January 20, 2020)

Dr Satchin Panda, The Circadian Code – Lose Weight, Supercharge your Energy and Sleep Well Every Night, 2018

Mel Robbins, The 5 Second Rule – Transform your Life, Work and Confidence with Everyday Courage, 2017

Gretchen Rubin, Better than Before – What I Learned About Making and Breaking Habits to Sleep More, Quit

Sugar, Procrastinate Less, and Generally Build a Happier Life, 2015

Iman Salem, Amy Ramser, Nancy Isham, and Mahmoud A. Ghannoum, "The Gut Microbiome as a Major Regulator of the Gut-Skin Axis", July 10, 2018, https://www.ncbi.nlm.nih.gov/pmc/articles/PMC6048199/ (accessed June 18, 2020)

S J Scott, Bad Habits No More: 25 Steps to Break and Bad Habit, 2015, Kindle Edition

Soil Association, "Why choose organic?", https://www.soilassociation.org/organic-living/why-organic (accessed August 26, 2020)

Justin and Erica Sonnenburg, Gut Reactions – How Healthy Insides Can Improve Your Weight, Mood and Wellbeing, 2015, Kindle Edition

World Health Organisation. "5 keys to a healthy diet.", https://www.who.int/nutrition/topics/5keys_healthydiet/en/ (accessed November 27, 2019)

World Health Organisation, "Noncommunicable Diseases", https://www.who.int/news-room/fact-sheets/detail/noncommunicable-diseases (accessed February 25, 2020)

ACKNOWLEDGMENTS

This book would not have been possible without the support of my family. A special thank you to Gavin, Evie, and Stuart, for their unique blend of love and sass. And to my parents who have given me the time and space needed to write this book.

Thank you to my audience at The Lifestyle Circle. I appreciate each and every one of you.

To Louise Thompson for her ninja coaching skills, and for helping me to make the transition. I am a wellbeing warrior!

Thanks to my editor, Tiffany Shand, for her expert eye and guidance.

Thanks to Latte Goldstein at River Design Books for my book cover design and his helpful advice throughout the process.

To everyone who has contributed their stories, thoughts, ideas, and opinions, and to those of you reading this now: Thank you!

ABOUT THE AUTHOR

Claire Hamilton is the founder of The Lifestyle Circle, an online platform dedicated to inspiring and empowering people to change their habits to get their best skin.

After a 17-year career in HR and People Development, and a 10-year struggle with her skin, Claire launched The Lifestyle Circle to contribute to the conversation we need to have about how we better manage skin conditions.

By raising awareness of the effects of skin issues, sharing stories, and highlighting what's working, Claire hopes that more people will find the relief they so desperately need.

Connect with Claire

www.thelifestylecircle.com

facebook.com/thelifestylecircle

pinterest.com/thelifestylecir

Printed in Great Britain
by Amazon